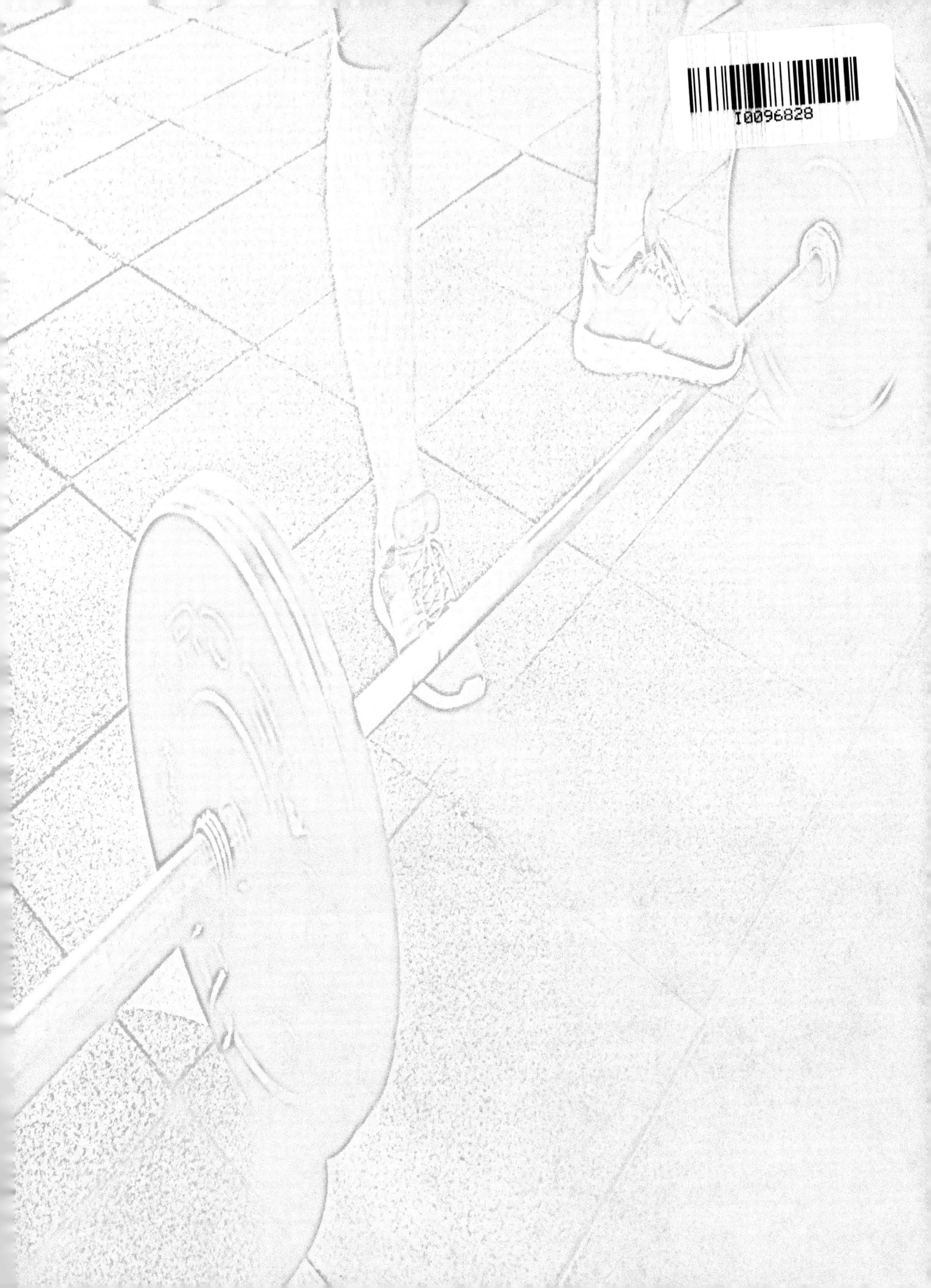

Resistance Band Workouts for Seniors

Beginner to Advanced Exercises to Improve Mobility, Bone Health and Muscle Strength After 60

Baz Thompson

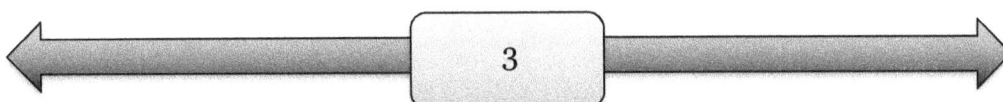

Table of Contents

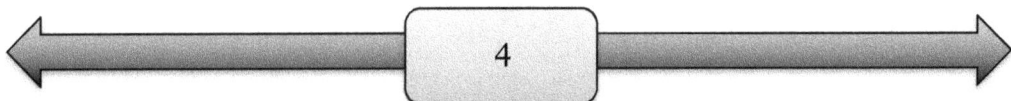

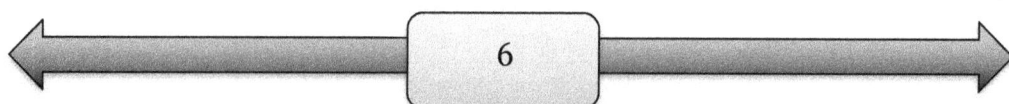

BEFORE YOU START READING

As a special gift, I included a logbook and my book, **"Strength Training After 40"**
(regularly priced at $16.97 on Amazon) and the best part is,
you get access to all of them for

FREE.

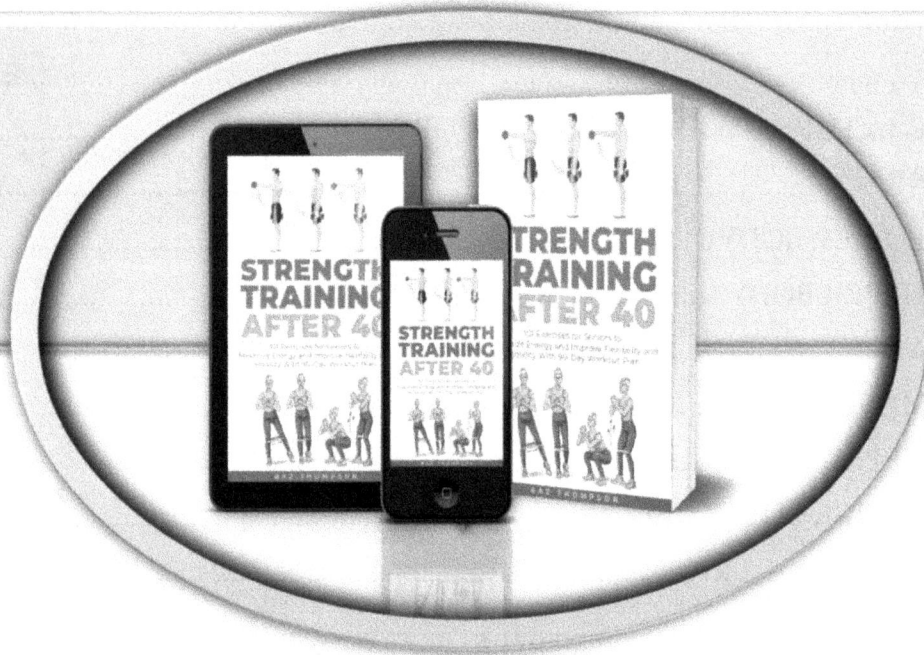

What's in it for me?

- 101 highly effective strength training exercises that can help you reach the highest point of your fitness performance
- Foundational exercises to improve posture and increase range of motion in your arms, shoulders, chest, and back
- Stretches to help you gain flexibility and find deep relaxation
- Workout Logbook to help you keep track of your accomplishments and progress. Log your progress to give you the edge you need to accomplish your goals.

SCAN ME

SCAN THE QR CODE

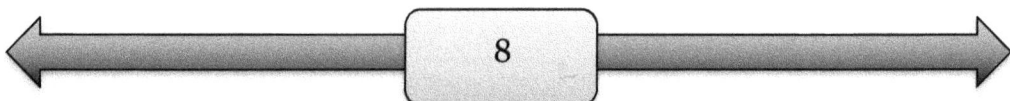

Introduction

Welcome to this fun and informative book about better health after 60! We will learn how resistance bands are a way to strengthen your bones and your muscles. Plus, workout programs are provided for you whatever your level of fitness, be it beginner, intermediate, or advanced.

Have you noticed as the years and decades go by that your joints are stiff, your muscles are losing mass, and your body has some mobility issues? It happens to all of us over time as we grow older. Perhaps you have extra challenges because of some bone loss or weakening through osteopenia or osteoporosis. Or you are recovering from surgery and trying to get your strength back so that you can return to doing the things you love. As we age, it becomes increasingly important to maintain and build our health so that we can not only stay active but also so we increase our chances of functioning independently. Daily tasks like personal care, dressing, preparing meals, walking up and down stairs, and driving are all dependent on our ability to do them on our own. According to the Centers for Disease Control (CDC), just over one-quarter of the U.S. adult population has some sort of disability. Of those adults, 11% have difficulty walking up and down stairs, and over 6% struggle to complete errands alone (Centers for Disease Control and Prevention, 2020).

I have seen this first-hand in my own life.

Personal Connection

My favorite uncle when I was growing up was my Uncle Jim. He wasn't really related to my parents, but was a long-time family friend that we all knew and loved. Uncle Jim was a carpenter that made everything from kitchen cabinets to baby changing tables. He was good at what he did and had a woodshop in the second garage on his property. Sometime during our childhood, all the boys in our family took turns helping Uncle Jim in his woodshop. We learned basic woodworking skills and messed up plenty of times along the way. He didn't get mad at our mistakes, but somehow turned them into learning lessons and a few laughs. I eventually moved away from my hometown to live and work in another city, but I carried with me the good memories and life lessons provided by Uncle Jim and his woodshop.

Several years later, I was visiting my hometown, family, and friends. I was surprised to learn that Uncle Jim was no longer working with wood. Granted, he was older and had lost his wife, so I decided to pay him a visit. When I went to his home, I was saddened by what I saw. Even though Uncle Jim greeted me with his famous crooked smile, I could see that his strength and vigor had deteriorated. He told me that a few years prior he had lost his balance and fallen off a ladder. The resulting broken pelvis and twisted ankle took nearly a year to heal and be functional again. He had a hard time going up and down the staircase to his garage, which is why he wasn't spending time in his woodshop. Uncle Jim felt that if he could strengthen his muscles and bones, he would be back to his old self. I took that as a challenge and gave him several exercises he could do right in his own home. Resistance bands, plus some other exercises that I tailored for him, helped him start to regain his strength. He is back to enjoying time in his beloved woodshop and working on small projects.

While this story has a happy ending, there are many similar stories out there that don't. People get injured, have surgery, lose strength, and eventually go downhill quickly in their health, their mood, and their outlook on life. So, what's the solution? From what I've seen, one of the keys to a successful outcome is improving bone health and muscle strength through simple exercises.

A Solution

You might be wondering how I helped my uncle recover and gain strength. One of the tools that I used was resistance bands. I have found these stretchy pieces of rubber or elastic are easy for people of all ages to use. They are lightweight, portable, and don't cost a lot. How do resistance bands help you to reclaim strength and maintain health? Well, you will see as we go through the book how they can specifically help certain areas of the body.

The top reasons for using resistance bands include their ease of use and the many options they provide to work the body. They are uncomplicated and greatly reduce your chance of injury, especially if you are just regaining balance, flexibility, and strength after an illness or surgery.

It is important to think about your motives for starting a program of exercises with resistance bands. To accomplish anything, you need a goal. What is your goal? Some possibilities might include

- gaining mobility in your arms, legs, and spine
- getting back in shape after an injury or surgery
- increasing the range of motion in your joints
- losing a little weight
- reducing back pain

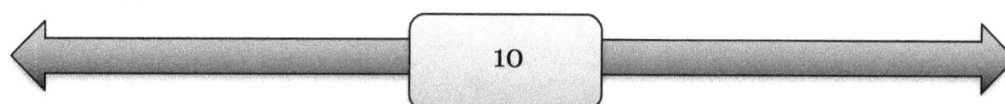

- rehabilitating a particular muscle or joint
- strengthening your abdominal and core muscles
- or you want to play with your grandkids without fear of straining something!

We all have different reasons for exercising. Identify yours. Your goal will help you find a plan that suits you, provide the motivation to get started, and above all, stick with the program until you see results.

How to Use This Book

Now that you have thought about and identified your "why" for embarking on an exercise program with resistance bands, let's talk about how you can use this book. I've written this book with you, the reader, in mind. My goal is to help you get to where you want to go, and in this case, it's the road to better health after 60. You can do it and I will show you how. Before you do anything else, please do me a favor. Check with your doctor or healthcare provider. I don't know each of your situations and medical challenges, so it is important that you consult with the medical professionals that do. They will be able to tell you what will work for you and what won't regarding an exercise plan. Take this book with you to your next doctor's visit and let them know you'd like to start on this program. Get their feedback and then go from there. Don't skip this step!
This book is divided up into three main sections.

- **Part 1: The Foundation**. The why and the what concerning resistance bands are talked about in Chapters 1 and 2, so you are educated on the tools you will be using. More importantly, you will learn what kinds of bands are available, the benefits of using them, and what precautions to look for.

- **Part 2: The Exercises.** All the different moves are explained in detail in this section. Chapter 3 contains exercises for the biceps and triceps', the workhorses of our arms. Our chest and back training are featured in Chapter 4 and will focus on the many muscles that help us to stand up tall. Chapter 5 is focused on the all-important core and glute muscles that support our torso. We concentrate on the quadriceps and hamstring leg muscles that get us walking in Chapter 6. The last chapter in this section, Chapter 7, is all about the forearms and calves which can sometimes be neglected.

- **Part 3: The Action Plan.** Here is where the fun begins! We have put together a series of one-week programs for you. Each one is tailored to your fitness level, whether it is beginner, intermediate, or advanced. Learn to do a week's exercises and increase in strength before moving on to the next level.

Thank you so much for downloading my book If you are enjoying the book so far, please leave me 4-5 rating on Amazon (You can always change if after reading the whole book). This will help many other people who are in the same situation as you find my book. Yor support means more to me than words can express.

Scan the QR code to leave a Rating

Are you ready to get started on your journey to increased bone density, stronger muscles, and better health?
Let's go!

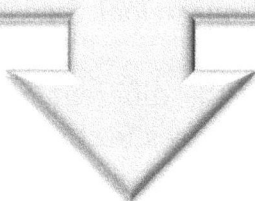

Part 1
The
Foundation

Chapter 1

The Equipment

You've probably seen them at the gym, the physical therapist, or your doctor's office. What are they? Resistance bands. Sometimes called exercise bands, resistance loops, resistance tubes, or therapy bands, these stretchy bands were invented in the late 19th or early 20th century. They were originally used for strengthening and expanding the chest. In the mid-20th century, resistance bands were employed by physical therapists to rehabilitate muscles after a patient's surgeries or injuries. Eventually, these bands crossed over from being used by doctors and therapists into use by athletes and physical fitness trainers to increase strength and training. Now, they are available to everyone and can be purchased at a variety of retail stores and online.

In this chapter, we look at why we should train with resistance bands and how that benefits us. We also go over the different types of bands (there are a lot of choices!) and which one is right for you.

Why Train with Resistance Bands

Resistance training is any type of exercise that uses resistant forces to strengthen muscles. Sometimes it is called strength training or weightlifting. Traditionally, resistance training involved lifting handheld free weights such as dumbbells or barbells. Weight machines at gyms achieve the same thing. Your muscles must work harder to lift heavy things and as a result, the muscle tissue breaks down and new tissue growth is stimulated. As a result, they become stronger. Another benefit of resistance training is that it builds bone density. The strain on your bones from lifting weight causes the older bone tissue to break down and kick-starts new bone tissue growth. Because of this, your bones become denser from the new growth.

What about resistance bands? They are an excellent way to participate in resistance training without having to purchase or store bulky weights. It can also be safer for those who are uncomfortable using handheld weights or lack grip strength. Do they work as well as traditional weights? Absolutely! Let's cover some of the benefits of using resistance bands.

- **Builds bone density:** As mentioned earlier, the strain or loading that happens in bones when engaged in resistance training helps the bones to rid themselves of old tissue and build new tissue, leading to greater bone denseness. Additionally, bones benefit from multi-directional movement, meaning not being loaded in the same direction each time. Resistance bands are great for this because they provide adaptive ways to move.
- **Convenient:** Resistance bands are the ultimate in convenience! Lightweight, portable, and inexpensive, they can be used at home or while traveling.

- **Easy on the joints:** Using resistance bands is easy on the joints, such as wrists, elbows, shoulders, hips, knees, and ankles. It's important to learn proper form and practice good techniques when doing any kind of resistance training.
- **Lowers body fat:** Studies have shown that exercising with resistance bands also lowers overall body fat and contributes to better body composition (Liu et al., 2022).
- **Increases muscle engagement:** The muscles are engaged to a greater degree because the resistance changes during the exercise. A common exercise goal is to "surprise" your muscles so that they don't adapt to the same movement and hit a plateau. Resistance bands can surprise your muscles throughout an exercise because as the band is stretched, the degree of resistance increases. This causes our muscles to adapt to how much force is needed because the workload has changed.
- **Strengthens muscles:** A recent study found that training with elastic bands was just as effective in building muscular strength as conventional methods, such as weights (Lopes et al., 2019).

These are a few of the common benefits of resistance band training. On top of all that, resistance bands are easy to use for anyone, regardless of age or strength. Next, we look at the different types of bands available.

Types of Resistance Bands

There are many different types of resistance bands. They come in different shapes, colors, lengths, and resistance levels. As a general rule of thumb, thinner and skinnier bands are used for smaller muscles like those in the arms. These cover more distance and can be moved more readily. Thicker and wider bands have less range and are used for larger muscles like those in the legs and lower body. Most bands can be divided into two overarching categories: flat or tubular.

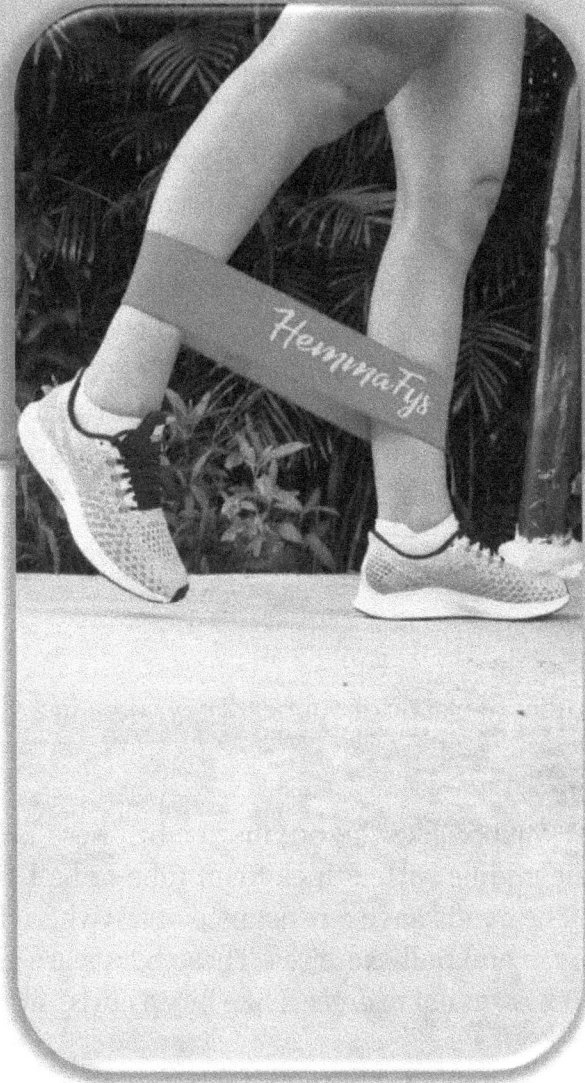

Flat Bands

The flat bands are flat pieces of rubber or elastic in a variety of thicknesses and lengths. These include

- **loop bands:** These look like big rubber bands. They are around 40 inches all the way around. In addition to being flat, they come in a variety of widths. The thinner the width of the band, the less resistance it will have. For instance, a band that is a one-half inch wide may have a resistance of anywhere from five to 25 pounds. Contrast this to a band that is two and one-half inches wide that can have a resistance of 60 to 170 pounds. These bands are great for full-body workouts, physical therapy, and stretching.

- **mini bands:** Similar to loop bands, mini bands are the smaller version. They are wider and shorter in length and are oftentimes covered in fabric to keep them from rolling over on themselves. Sometimes they are called booty bands because of their frequent use in exercises that involve the glutes. These bands are great for hip and glute activation exercises and toning in that area as well as leg extensions.

- **therapy bands:** These bands are the lightest, longest, and thinnest of the flat bands. They are not loops but are free bands, meaning they are long strips of elastic that can be used for a variety of exercises. Some of them can be over six feet long! They are frequently used for physical therapy and Pilates workouts because they have lower resistance, between three and 10 pounds. These bands are especially good for those who are just starting out with resistance bands or those who are recovering from injury.

Tubular Bands

These bands are hollow tubes of elastic or rubber. They come in a variety of thicknesses and lengths. These include

- **Figure 8 bands:** Shaped like the number eight, these bands are tubes that have been secured in the middle with a thick foam tube or ball and have handles at both ends of the eight. The bands have a resistance of anywhere from eight to 20 pounds and are used for push and pull exercises. These bands are great for side-to-side and forward/backward movement exercises like bicep curls, sit ups, and side lunges.

- **tube bands with handles:** These are popular at gyms and physical therapist offices. They consist of a long elastic tube that has handles on both ends. The resistance level depends on the thickness of the tube and can be from five to 50 pounds. Thicker tubes have more resistance and thinner ones have less. Because of their handles, these tubes can be anchored on one end to a door or chair to provide alternative ways to use the bands. These bands are great for exercises that require pulling, such as bicep curls, or pushing, such as overhead shoulder presses.

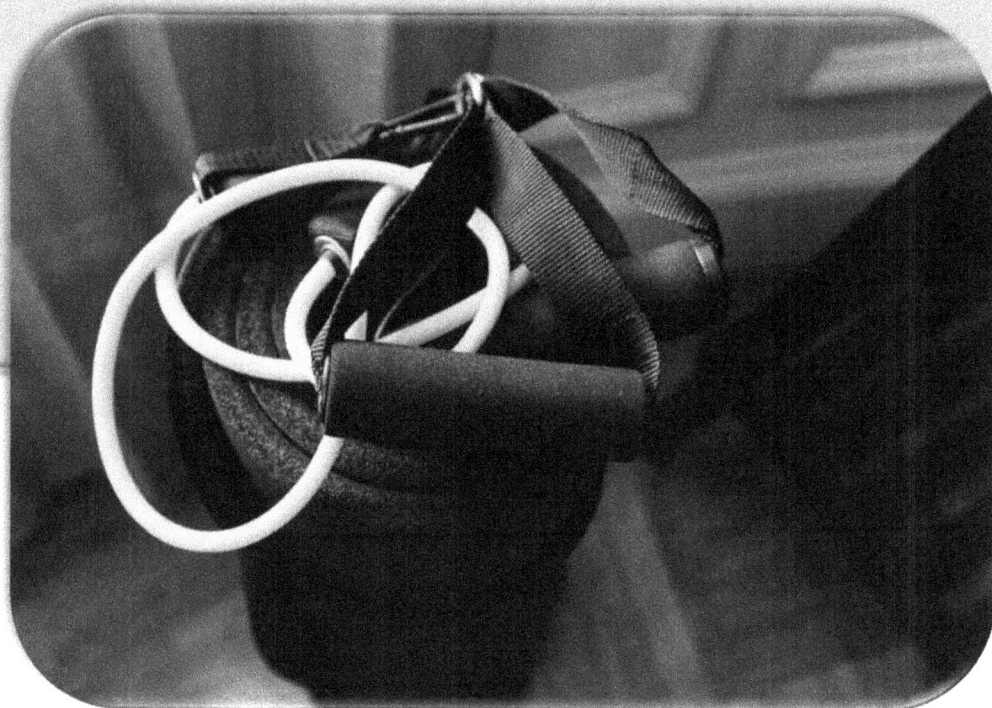

Which Resistance Band is Right for You?

Now that you have learned about the five main types of resistance bands, how do you choose the one that is right for you? There are several things to consider including

- **accessories:** If you do exercises that need an anchor point, consider getting bands that can be attached to accessories like ankle cuffs, door attachments, or handles.

- **material:** The thinnest therapy bands are made of rubber and are great upper body moves, stretching, or for beginners just starting out with band exercises. But this type isn't always ideal for some exercises because of their tendency to roll up. For lower body moves like squats and side shuffles, a fabric-covered band works better.

- **price point:** Bands are available in all price ranges! For the most part, they are easy on the budget and easy to find in stores or online. Look for a good quality band from a reputable manufacturer or store.

- **resistance level:** As mentioned previously, usually the thinner the band, the less resistance, and vice versa. For those just beginning to exercise again, go with a thinner and easier resistance level and work your way up as you gain strength. If you are already active and exercise regularly, you may be ready for a thicker, higher-resistance band.

Still not sure what to buy? My recommendation is to try out several different types of bands at your local gym or therapist's office. See what is comfortable for you at your given fitness level. Most likely, no one here is training for the Olympics, so don't be ashamed or worried about what others think regarding what band you are using. Use the one that makes sense for you. If you are purchasing, start with one band such as a therapy band, loop band, or tube band with handles, and get used to using it. Over time, you will probably accumulate more than one band, because they are all slightly different and you will want some variety in your routines.

Action Items for Chapter 1

Now that you know the benefits of resistance bands and the five types that are most common, it's time to take action!

1. Choose which type of band you are going to start out with. Will it be one band or a set of bands so you can level up when you are ready?
2. Look in stores and online for the band(s) you want and identify one that fits your need for accessories, material, price point, and resistance level. Then, purchase it!

Chapter 2
The Technique

Every exercise and every sport require that the athlete know and practice good technique. Resistance band exercises are no different. It is important that you learn the best way to use them so that you will get the maximum benefit from the work you are putting into it! The proper technique will also help minimize the chance of injury to yourself. In this chapter, we look at what good form looks like and how to practice proper breathing. We also identify common mistakes to avoid and discuss care tips for your bands. Finally, we learn how to put together a program that will help you achieve your fitness goals.

Good Form

What is good form? In exercise, practicing good form means performing the exercise as directed by following directions and precautions. Exercise directions normally are designed to incorporate efficient body mechanics that ensure things are moving correctly and to your benefit. Good form doesn't mean perfection (because that is never possible) but it does mean being efficient and safe.

Some characteristics of good form when using resistance bands include

- **control:** Your movements are not herky-jerky or out of control. You should maintain control of the band and your body from the start to the finish of the exercise movement. If you find that you aren't able to move with intention and control, consider going with a less resistant band or performing the move without a band until you master it.
- **focus:** The mind-muscle connection is real! Think about each move you are doing and what muscle you are working. Just going through the motions while your mind drifts and thinks about something else is not doing your fitness any good. By staying present in the moment, actively thinking about the exercise, and watching what your body is currently doing, your muscle activation increases and so do the results.
- **good posture:** Standing up straight with your shoulders back and tummy tucked in is a good starting point for any exercise. Maintaining a tight core during exercise helps to protect your back and keep your balance. Good posture also helps you get the most out of your workout because the mechanics of your body are working as they should.
- **proper breathing:** It's natural to hold your breath during exertion, but don't do it! Proper breathing through an exercise means inhaling as you start the movement and exhaling at the place of most resistance. Inhale again as you return to the starting position. Believe it or not, good breathing techniques can protect your back and strengthen your core as you move through the exercises.

- **rest:** Take a short break between exercises. This rest can be anywhere from a few seconds to a minute or longer, depending on what your body requires. Jumping from exercise to exercise without any breaks doesn't give you a chance to catch your breath and reset your focus for the next move. These micro-recovery moments are important to your good form.
- **warm-up:** Don't skip the warm-up! Exercising cold doesn't give your body a chance to loosen up and prepare. Taking five to ten minutes to walk or move your body and get the blood moving to your extremities makes a difference in how your body responds to the strength training you will be doing. Muscles that have not been warmed up and prepped for exercise are more likely to suffer injury.

Common Mistakes

There are some mistakes that folks commonly make when they are just starting out using resistance bands. Even seasoned gym rats that have used them a long time can make these missteps, too. These common mistakes include

- **allowing slack in the band:** From the start to the end of each exercise, there should be tension in the band. From the starting point, the band tension should be minimal (meaning no loose-goosey band!) and increase in resistance as you perform the movement.
- **anchoring them improperly:** Some bands allow you to anchor them to an object such as a door or sturdy piece of furniture. Choose an anchor point that is smooth with no sharp edges that could damage the band and one that is immovable so that you don't risk it moving or releasing the band and injuring you.
- **using a band with too little resistance:** The band you choose for your exercise should have enough resistance for you to complete the move. Bands should not be stretched over two times their length. This may cause the band to release while at its maximum tension and snap back at you.
- **using a band that has too much resistance:** Choosing a band that is too strong and stiff can result in you having to yank on it too hard and lead to improper form. You increase the chances of injuring yourself when you sacrifice good form. You should be able to perform the full range of motion required for the exercise without jerking or yanking.
- **using a damaged or weakened band:** Quality-made bands are made of good materials and will last a long time. However, they do occasionally get damaged or weakened in some areas. Discard damaged bands and replace them with new ones.
- **using the wrong type of band for the exercise you are performing:** It's good to have more than one type of band to perform full-body workouts. Mini bands, or booty bands, are great for exercises involving the glutes and the lower half of your

body but aren't as well suited for bicep curls. Choose the band appropriate for the area of the body and the exercise you will be performing.

Care Tips

Once you have purchased the resistance band or set of bands that will work for you, take the extra step to store and care for them properly so that they last you a long time. These bands are pretty indestructible at first, but they do deteriorate over time. Bands should be replaced as they become damaged or after having owned them for a couple of years. Some band care tips include

- always check bands before you use them for cuts, flaws, and nicks in the elastic or rubber that can compromise the safety of the band. If the band has handles, check that these are securely attached and not fraying where they are attached.
- not using soap or cleaners on the bands as these can interact with the elastic or rubber and break them down. Certain cleaning agents will weaken the bands, so it is best to wipe them down with a clean sponge or cloth that has been dampened with water only.
- storing the bands in a clean, dry place away from extreme cold or heat, which can weaken the elastic or rubber. Do not store them in direct sunlight or near a source of heat.

Putting a Program Together

Let's start on the fun stuff: putting together an exercise program! All this knowledge you are gaining helps you only if you put it into action. But you might be thinking, "Wait, I don't know how to make a workout program." We will be learning how to do that in this section. So, what components are necessary for a good program?

- **Define a goal:** Remember we touched on this in the Introduction? What is your goal? I know guys, you want bigger biceps because we all do. But seriously, think about what you want to achieve with these exercises. Leg strength to go up and down stairs easily? Arm and back strength to lift grandkids up and onto your lap? Core and abdominal strength to carry groceries from your car to your kitchen counter? Or maybe you just want to get fit and lose a few pounds.
- **Identify exercises:** Pinpoint the exercises that will help you reach your goal. For example, if you want to have stronger arms and grip strength, then your target will be exercises that build your forearms, biceps, shoulders, and triceps. If your goal is overall better health, then you'll want to include exercises that are full-body to incorporate all the muscle groups.

- **Set a schedule:** How many days a week can you devote to working out? Be realistic. When you are just starting out, you won't want to overdo it and schedule yourself five days a week. Start off with a conservative two workouts per week as recommended by experts (U.S. Department of Health and Human Services, 2018). Resistance band exercises are strength training and should be spaced out with days of cardio or rest days in between. Think about if you are also doing other strength training with dumbbells or weight machines. You can piggyback and add some resistance band training on your weight training days or alternate them with each other.
- **Do it:** The best-laid plans are for naught if you don't actually follow through with them. Decide in advance that this is part of your life and what you do in order to maintain good health. So, like brushing your teeth, showering, and eating, exercising is part of what you do to take care of yourself.
- **Muscle recovery:** Be sure to leave days for muscle recovery. Delayed onset of muscle soreness (DOMS) may cause you to think that you are good to go, but the same muscles should not be trained every day. There is a difference between common muscle fatigue or soreness and true pain resulting from a strain or muscle injury.

In Part 3 of this book, we've included some workout programs for you as examples. Try these on for size, then adapt them or use them as a template for your own program.

Action Items for Chapter 2

Alright, are you ready to put into practice what you've learned in this chapter? Your action items now include

1. check with your doctor if you haven't already. Get their input and suggestions on what exercises are safe and appropriate for you and your current state of health.
2. keeping your goal in mind, identify what types of exercises will help you achieve your goal. You don't need to know the exercises yet; we cover that in the next few chapters. Put a tentative plan together that is realistic but still challenging.

Part 2 The Exercises

Chapter 3
Biceps and Triceps

The main muscles in your upper arms are the biceps and triceps. These muscles help you to do many daily tasks and activities. The bicep muscles are on the front of your upper arm and allow your arm to flex, bend in, and pull items to you. They make up about 30% of the muscle mass in your upper arm. The triceps are on the back of your upper arm and allow you to extend your arm down and push things away from you. These triceps muscles account for around 55% of the muscle mass in your upper arm (Holzbaur et al., 2007). So, you can see that strengthening these two muscle groups is important for arm strength and mobility!

Important terms to know include

- **rep**: This means a repetition or completing the exercise one time. Most exercises here will call for 10 reps.
- **set**: Once you have done the 10 reps, that is called a set. You will start off doing two sets and increase as you get stronger.

Let's get started!

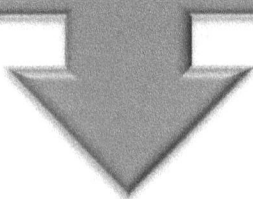

Bicep Exercises

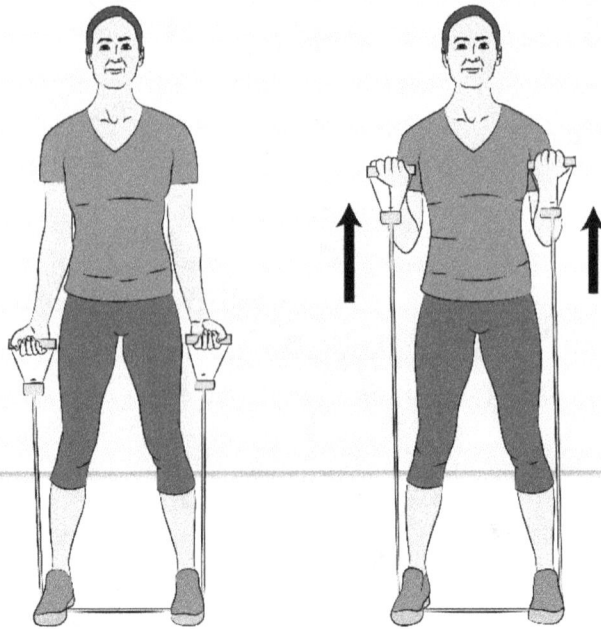

BICEP CURL

BAND USED: TUBE BANDS WITH HANDLES OR FIGURE 8 BAND |
TIME NEEDED: 3 MINUTES

DIRECTIONS:

1. Stand with your feet hip-width apart. Place the middle of the band under the middle of your feet and stand on it firmly.
2. Hold handles in each hand with your arms down along your sides. The band should not have any slack. If it does, loop the band around your hands once or find a shorter band.
3. Inhale, then bring both hands up with palms facing you as you bend your arms at the elbows. Exhale as your hands reach toward your shoulders.
4. Inhale as you slowly lower your hands back to the starting position. That is one rep.
5. Do 10 reps for 2 sets.

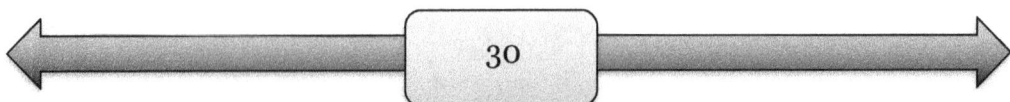

Make this harder by moving your feet wider apart to increase the resistance. You can also do this by changing to a thicker band. Need this to be easier? Stand with your feet closer together.

Take Care
Keep your wrists taut and don't allow them to bend or flop open.
Keep your upper arms close to your sides
as you perform the exercise.

SEE IT: youtu.be/LI1p31gp_fU

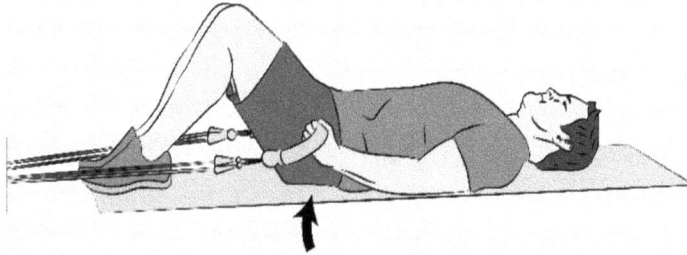

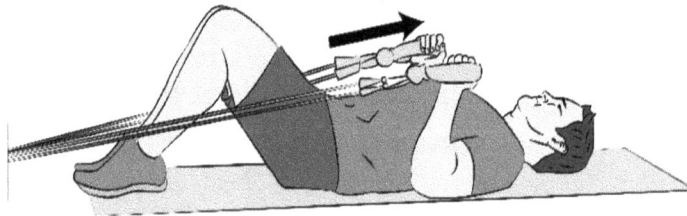

LYING HAMMER CURL

BAND USED: TUBE BANDS WITH HANDLES AND ANCHOR POINT |
TIME NEEDED: 3 MINUTES

DIRECTIONS:

1. Attach the middle of the tube band to a sturdy anchor point such as a door or couch. Lie down on your back with the anchor point just beyond your feet. Alternatively, you can loop the band under the bottom of your feet.
2. Hold on to the handles in each hand with your palms facing inward toward each other. Inhale then bend your elbows and bring your hands toward your shoulders and exhale as they are at their closest. Inhale as you return your hands to the starting position. This is one rep.
3. Do 10 reps for 2 sets.

Increase the resistance by moving farther away from the anchor point or looping the band around your hands once or twice.

Take Care:
The back of your arms should remain touching the floor as you move through the hammer curl.

SEE IT: bodylastics.com/exercise/lying-hammer-curl-with-bands-arms-down/

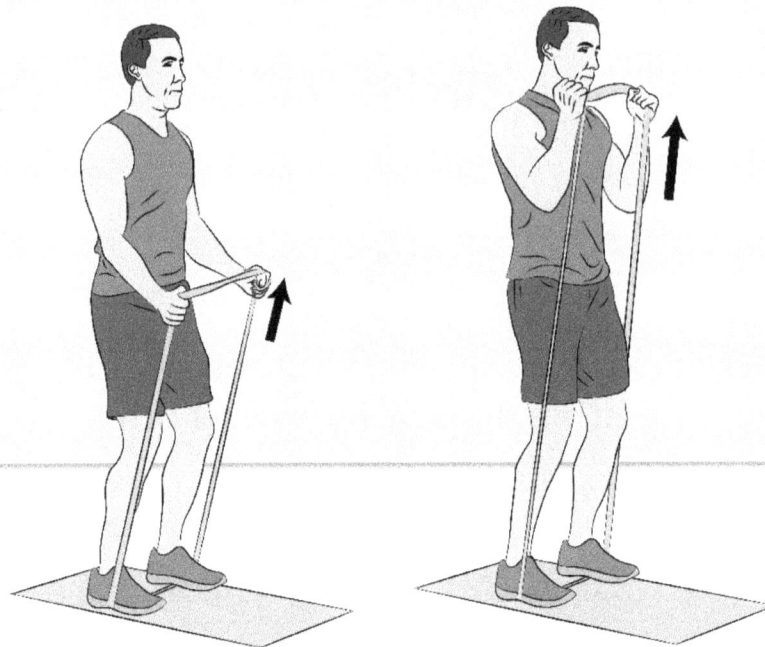

REVERSE BICEP CURL

BAND USED: LARGE LOOP BAND | **TIME NEEDED:** 3 MINUTES

DIRECTIONS:

1. Stand with feet hip-width distance apart and place one end of the loop under both feet. Hold the other end of the loop with both hands' palms down hip-width apart and resting on the front of your hips.
2. Inhale then bend your arms at the elbows and raise your hands up with knuckles facing the sky. Exhale as your hands reach the top of the movement near your shoulders, then inhale as you slowly lower your hands to the starting position. This is one rep.

3. Do 10 reps for 2 sets.

LEVEL UP:

For more intensity, move your feet farther apart to increase the resistance.

Take Care
Be sure that you keep your wrists level and taut as you perform this exercise. Don't let them bend or
flop down.

SEE IT: setforset.com/blogs/news/bicep-exercises-and-workouts-with-resistance-bands

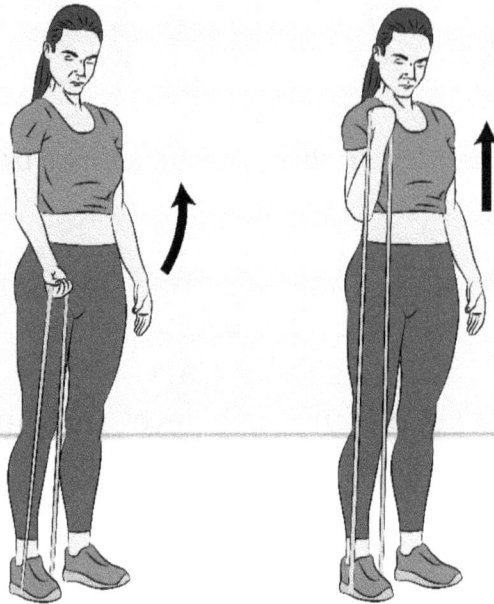

SINGLE ARM HAMMER CURL

BAND USED: FIGURE 8 BAND OR LARGE LOOP BAND |
TIME NEEDED: 4 MINUTES

DIRECTIONS:

1. Stand with feet hip-width distance apart. Loop one end of the band under your right foot. Hold the other end of the loop in your right hand with your palm facing toward the middle and your wrist in a neutral position.
2. Inhale then bend your elbow and bring your hand up so that your thumb moves toward your shoulder. Exhale as your hand reaches the top, then inhale as you lower your hand back to the starting position. This is one rep on the right side.
3. Do 10 reps for 2 sets on your right arm. Switch feet and arms and repeat on the left for 10 reps and 2 sets.

You may find you need heavier resistance with hammer curls because they work an additional muscle that isn't used in regular bicep curls. So, you have more muscle power and may need more resistance. Use a thicker band or loop it once more around your foot.

Take Care
Don't use momentum to swing your arm up or let it flop back down. Keep the movement controlled throughout the whole exercise.

SEE IT: hevyapp.com/exercises/hammer-curl-resistance-band/

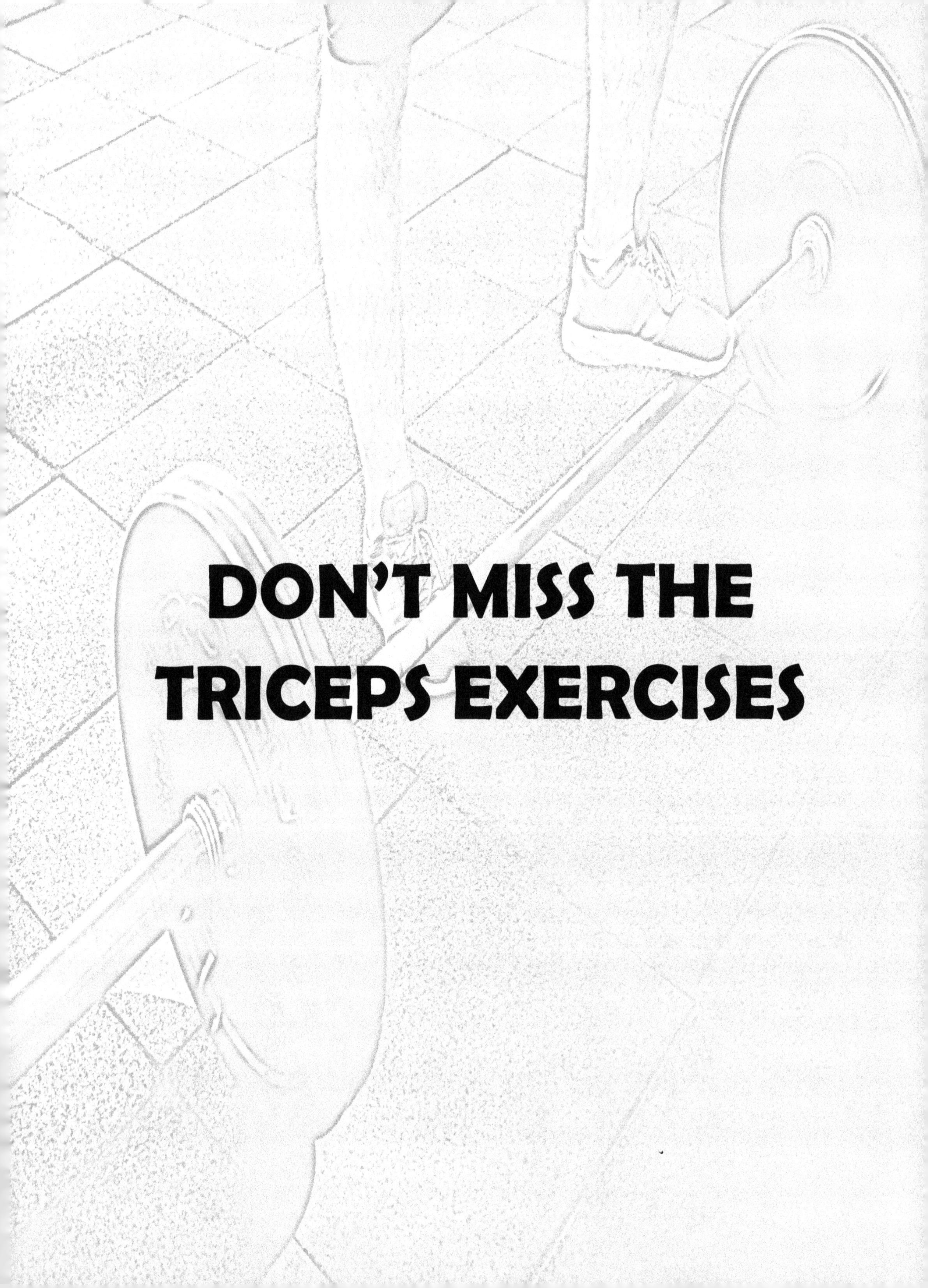

DON'T MISS THE TRICEPS EXERCISES

Triceps Exercises

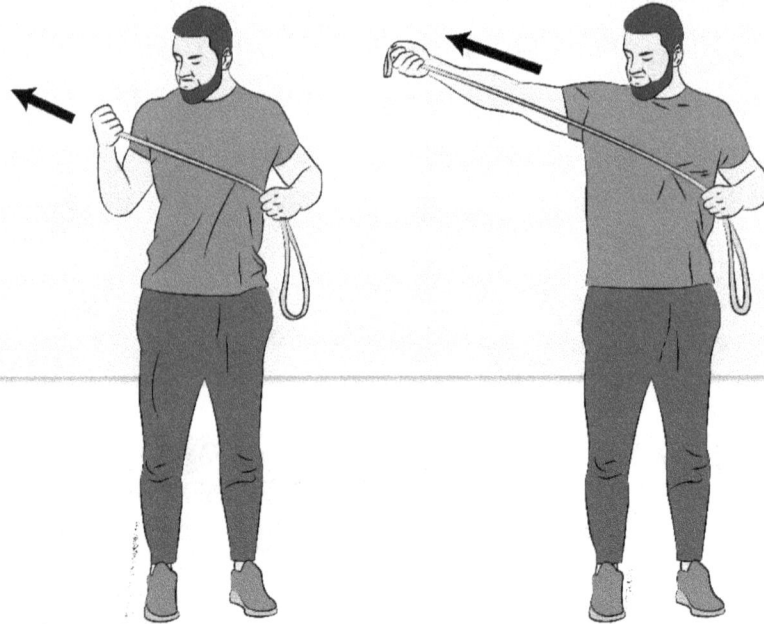

CROSSBOW TRICEP EXTENSION

BAND USED: LOOP BAND OR THERAPY BAND | **TIME NEEDED:** 4 MINUTES

DIRECTIONS:

1. Stand with feet hip-width distance apart. Hold one end of the band in your left hand and place your left fist on the outside of your lower ribs with knuckles facing up and palm down.
2. Hold the other end of the band with your right hand to where it is taut. Your right palm should be facing up to the sky.
3. Bend your elbow and move your right hand close to your right shoulder. Inhale as you straighten your right arm outwards and to the side of your body so that your right

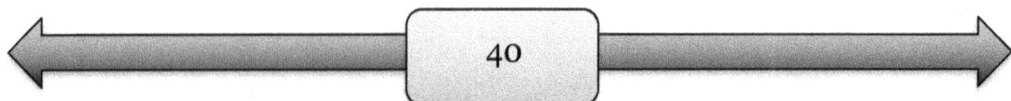

hand is the same height as your shoulder. Exhale as you squeeze your right tricep, then inhale as you return your hand to the starting position. This is one rep.

4. Do 10 reps for 2 sets on the right side. Switch arms and repeat on the left.

LEVEL UP:

You can make this exercise more challenging just by changing where you grip the band and increasing the resistance.

Take Care:
This exercise can also be done seated if desired.
Sit on a sturdy chair with feet flat on the floor and hip-width distance apart.

SEE IT: setforset.com/blogs/news/resistance-band-triceps-exercises

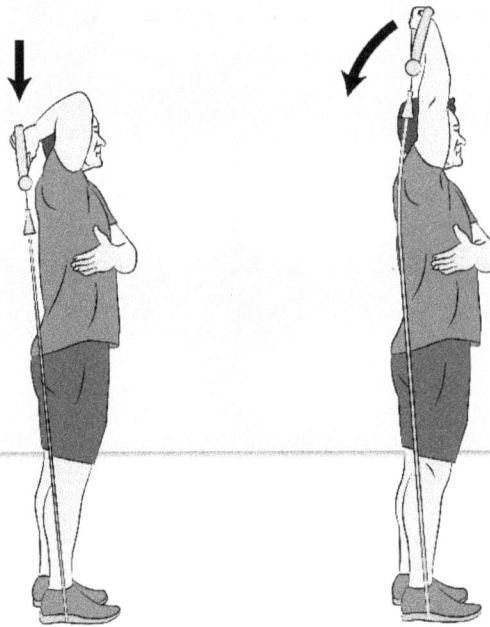

OVERHEAD TRICEP EXTENSION

BAND USED: LOOP BAND OR TUBE BAND WITH HANDLES | **TIME NEEDED:** 4 MINUTES

DIRECTIONS:

1. Stand with feet hip-width distance apart. Loop one end of the band under your right foot and stand on it firmly. Grasp the other end of the loop or handle with your right hand. Bend your right elbow and raise it so that it is pointing straight up above your head. Your right hand should be behind your right shoulder and pointing down.

2. Inhale as you straighten your right arm and bring your right hand straight up above you. Exhale as it reaches the top. Inhale as you slowly bend your elbow and carefully lower your right hand behind you toward your shoulder. This is one rep.

3. Do 10 reps for 2 sets on the right side. Switch to your left foot and left arm and repeat.

To make this more difficult, use a thicker band for more resistance. You can also do this with both hands at the same time.

Take Care

Be aware of your wrists. Keep them steady and don't allow them to bend back.

SEE IT: bodylastics.com/exercise/one-arm-overhead-triceps-extension-with-bands/

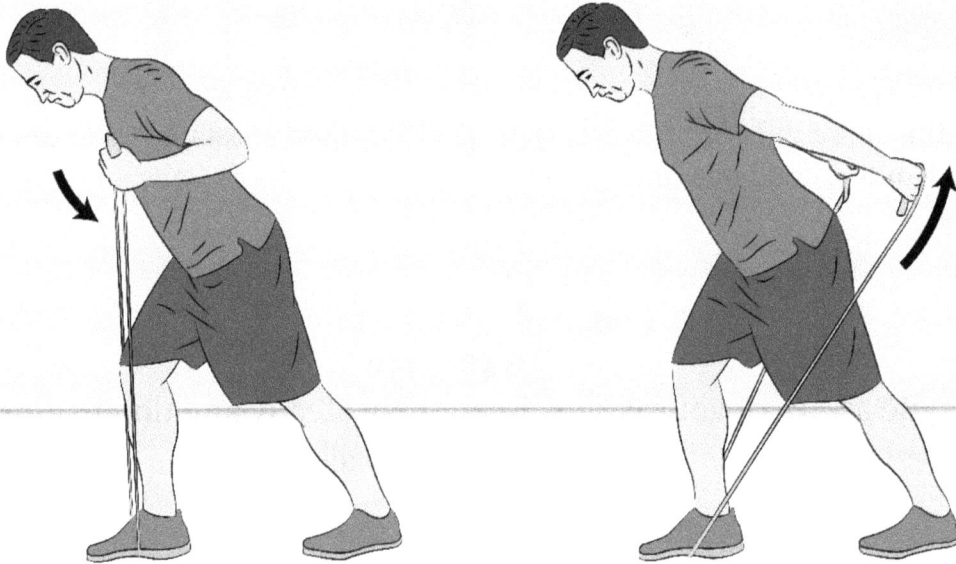

TRICEP KICKBACK

BAND USED: TUBE BAND WITH HANDLES | **TIME NEEDED:** 3 MINUTES

DIRECTIONS:

1. Place feet hip-width distance apart. Step the right foot forward so that the feet are now staggered. Loop the middle of the tube band under the right foot.
2. Bend the right knee and slightly lean your body forward over that knee.
3. Hold the handles of the band in each hand and bend your elbows as you bring your hands up to either side of your chest.
4. Inhale and, while keeping your elbows where they are, straighten your arms so that your hands are now behind you. Exhale as you squeeze your shoulder blades together

and fully extend your arms. Inhale and return your hands to the starting position. This is one rep.

5. Do 10 reps for 2 sets. Switch feet between sets.

LEVEL UP:

Make this more difficult by switching to a thicker band or by looping the band once under your foot to increase the resistance.

Take Care:
If you have balance issues, leaning forward may pose a problem. You can do one arm at a time and use your free hand to steady Yourself with a sturdy chair or countertop.

SEE IT: skimble.com/exercises/57597-band-tricep-kickback-how-to-do-exercise

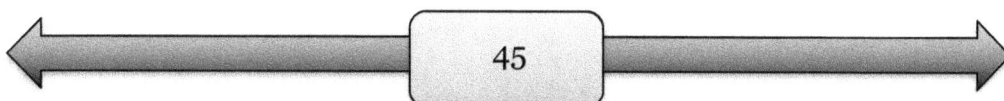

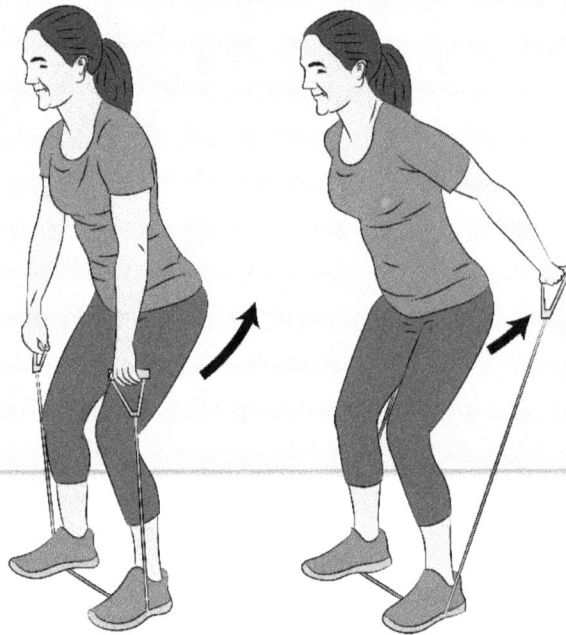

TRICEP SHOULDER PRESS

BAND USED: TUBE BAND WITH HANDLES | **TIME NEEDED:** 3 MINUTES

DIRECTIONS:

1. Stand with feet hip-width distance apart. Place the middle of the band under both feet and step on it firmly. Grab handles in each hand and face your palms to the back behind you. Keep your arms straight and close to the sides of your body.
2. Keep a slight bend in your knees and hinge forward at your hips. Inhale, then move your hands back and up behind you as far as you can. Exhale as you squeeze at the farthest point, then inhale as you return your hands to the starting position. This is one rep.
3. Do 10 reps for 2 sets.

By moving your feet wider apart, you can make this exercise more challenging. You can also loop the band around your hands once more to increase resistance.

Take Care
Don't get this confused with the triceps kickback.
The elbows are not bent in this exercise. They stay straight and Extended the whole time. Keep your neck long and loose so you don't hunch up your shoulders.

SEE IT: gethealthyu.com/exercise/resistance-band-triceps-shoulder-press/

"Good Will"

Helping others without expectation of anything in return has been proven to lead to increased happiness and satisfaction in life.

I would love to give you the chance to experience that same feeling during your reading experience today.

All it takes is a few moments of your time to answer one simple question:

Would you make a difference in the life of someone you've never met—without spending any money or seeking recognition for your good will?

If so, I have a small request for you.

If you've found value in your reading or listening experience today, I humbly ask that you take a brief moment right now to leave an honest review of this book. It won't cost you anything but 30 seconds of your time—just a few seconds to share your thoughts with others.

SCAN THE QR CODE

Your voice can go a long way in helping someone else find the same inspiration and knowledge that you have.

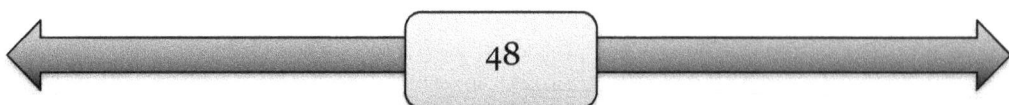

Chapter 4
Chest and Back

There are many benefits to strengthening your chest and back muscles. The muscles in these areas help to hold your body erect and keep a good posture. This is important for your lungs and better breathing. It is also a way to protect your spine and reduce stiffness and tension in your upper body. When you do strength training in your upper body, you are contributing to the efficiency of these muscles so they can continue to assist you in your daily life. Everyday tasks like carrying a bag of groceries, lifting up pets, opening doors, or even unscrewing the tops off of jars all require strength and mobility in our upper bodies.

Let's work these muscles

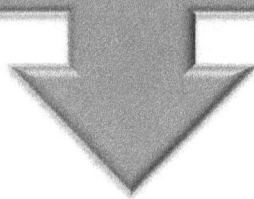

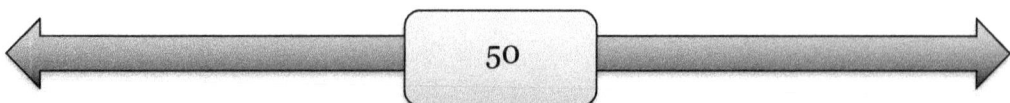

Chest Exercises

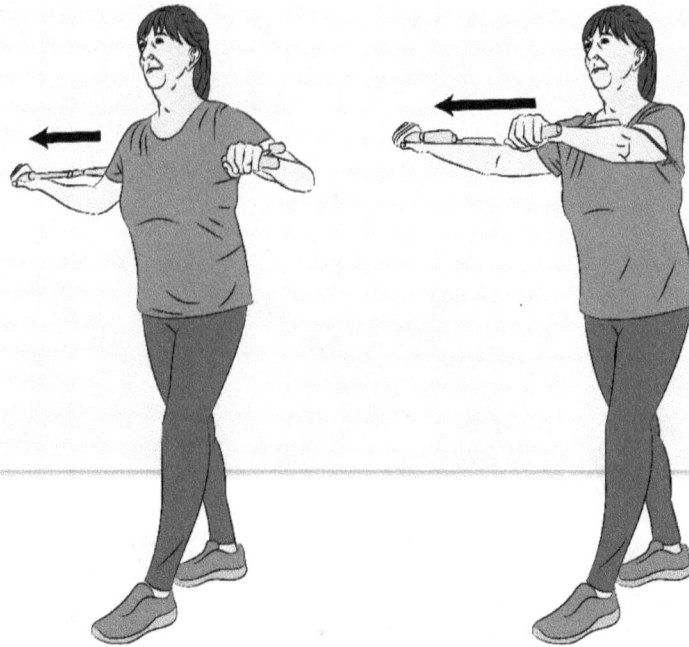

CHEST PUNCH

BAND USED: TUBE BAND WITH HANDLES | **TIME NEEDED:** 3 MINUTES

1. Stand with feet in a split stance. Place one foot slightly in front of the other and hip-width apart.
2. Loop the band around your body with the middle of the band in the middle of your upper back. Hold the handles in each hand with the band on the outside of your upper arms. Bring your hands up to shoulder height with your elbows bent and out to the sides.

3. Inhale then press both hands in front of you with palms facing front. Exhale as you extend elbows straight but don't lock them. Inhale as you slowly return your hands to starting position. That is one rep.
4. Do 10 reps for 2 sets. Switch forward foot between sets.

LEVEL UP:

Increase the intensity by looping the band once around your hands for extra resistance. Try pressing one arm at a time while holding the other one at shoulder height.

Take Care:
Make sure that the band doesn't roll up your back and onto your neck. If this happens, you can place the band, so it goes under your armpits rather than on the outside of your upper arms to help keep it in place.

SEE IT: youtu.be/SYVotAbHHpE

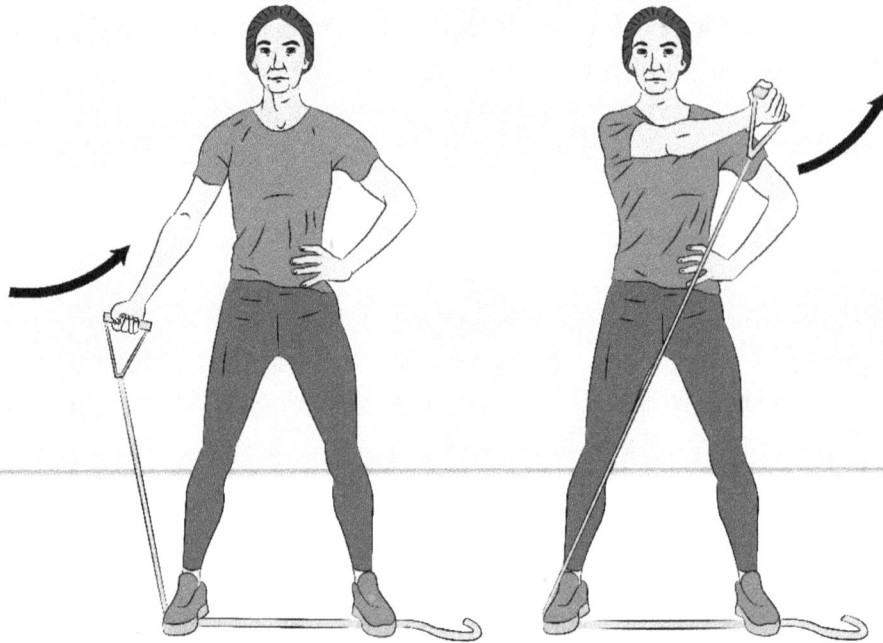

CROSSOVER FLY

BAND USED: TUBE BAND WITH HANDLES | **TIME NEEDED:** 4 MINUTES

DIRECTIONS:

1. Stand with feet hip-width distance apart. Place the middle of the band under your right foot as an anchor point.
2. Grab the handle that is closest to your right hand. The band should be taut with no slack. Your palm should be facing front in an underhand grip.
3. Inhale as you raise your right arm and hand up away from the right side of your body and cross it over diagonally so that your hand is now straight in front of your left shoulder. Don't bend your arm, but keep it straight. Exhale as you squeeze your right

chest muscle at the top of the move, then inhale as you return your arm to the starting position. This is one rep.

4. Do 10 reps for 2 sets. Switch to the other foot and arm and repeat.

LEVEL UP:

Make this more difficult by widening your stance to increase the resistance.

Take Care
Be sure not to twist your torso as you do this exercise.
You are working the pectoral muscles in your chest, so keep
your core tight and stable.

SEE IT: healthline.com/health/fitness/resistance-band-chest-workout

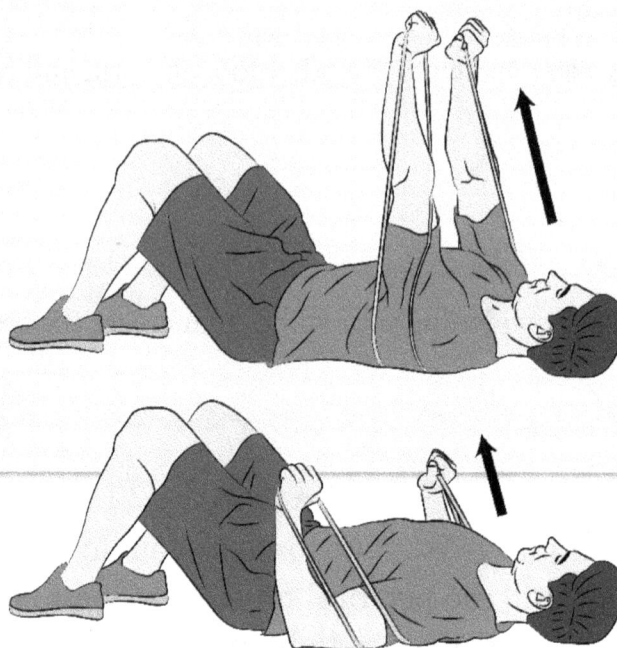

LYING CHEST PRESS

BAND USED: TUBE BAND WITH HANDLES | **TIME NEEDED:** 3 MINUTES

DIRECTIONS:

1. Lie down on the floor or on an exercise mat with your back on the ground. Put the middle of the band under your upper back toward the bottom of your shoulder blades. Hold on to the handles in each hand and bend your elbows so that they are at shoulder height on either side of your body and touching the floor. Your upper arm from shoulder to elbow should be resting on the floor.

2. Inhale then press your hands up toward the ceiling as you straighten your arms. Exhale as your hands touch and you squeeze your chest muscles. Inhale as you bring your arms back to the starting position. This is one rep.

3. Do 10 reps for 2 sets.

LEVEL UP:

Increase the resistance and make this more challenging by looping the band around your hands. You can also switch to a thicker band.

Take Care:
Don't allow your hands to raise higher than shoulder height. Keep them at chest level throughout the exercise to protect your shoulders.

SEE IT: freetrainers.com/exercise/exercise/bands_lying_chest_press/

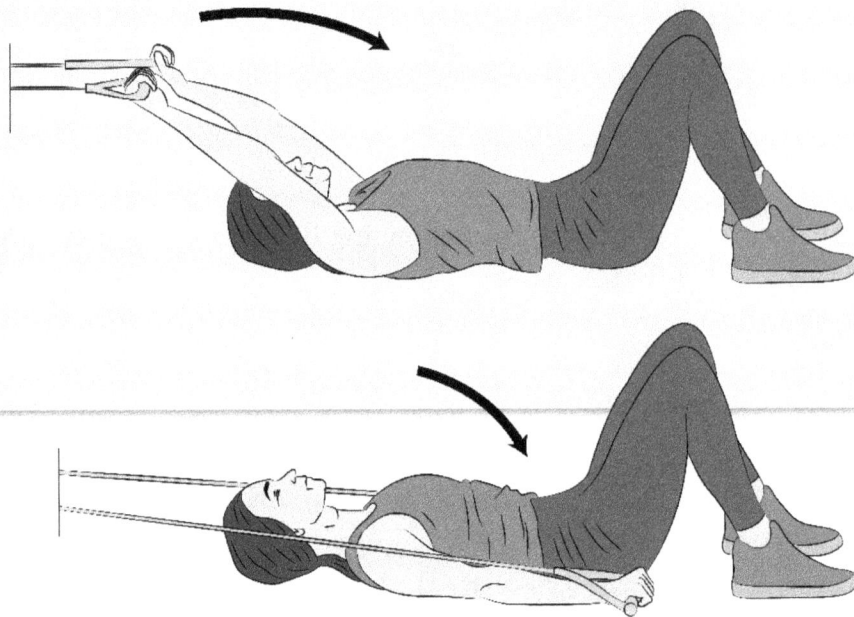

PULLOVER

BAND USED: TUBE BAND WITH HANDLES | **TIME NEEDED:** 3 MINUTES

DIRECTIONS:

1. Loop the band around a heavy piece of furniture or immovable object at floor level. Lie down on your back with the anchor point behind you and above your head.
2. Bend your knees so that they are pointing up to the sky and your feet are flat on the floor. Grab the handles of the band with your palms facing up. Your arms should be straight up over your head and touching the floor.
3. Inhale then bring both hands and arms up toward the sky and pull them down to your hips. Exhale as your hands approach your hips, palms down. Inhale as you reverse the motion and bring your arms back to the starting position. This is one rep.

4. Do 10 reps for 2 sets.

LEVEL UP:

To make this more challenging, face your palms out from either side of your body as you bring them down toward your hips.

Take Care
Ensure that you are anchoring to an object that is not going to move and possibly injure you when you pull down.

SEE IT: healthline.com/health/fitness/resistance-band-chest-workout

DON'T MISS THE BACK EXERCISES

Back Exercises

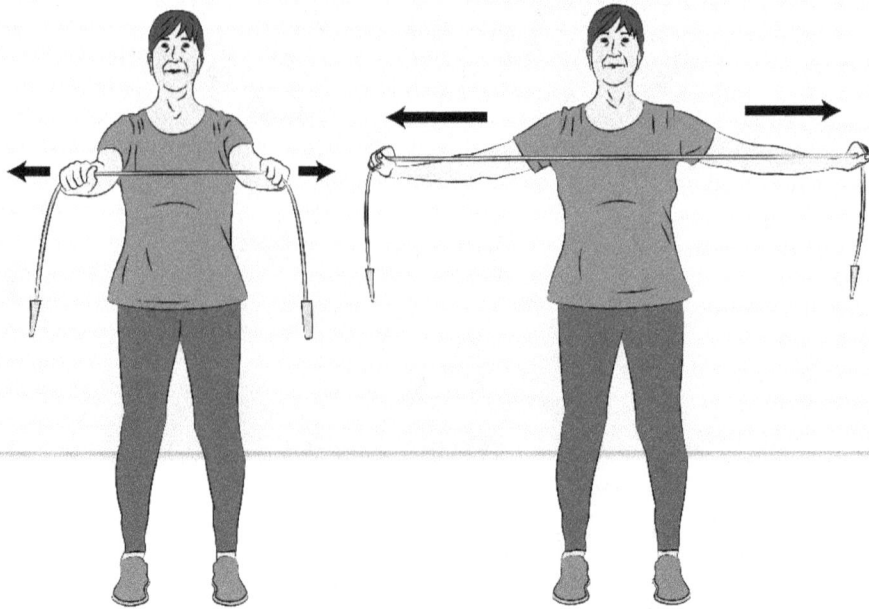

PULL APART

BAND USED: THERAPY BAND OR TUBE BAND WITH HANDLES | **TIME NEEDED:** 3 MINUTES

DIRECTIONS:

1. Stand with feet hip-width distance apart. Hold the band with both hands about hip-width distance apart and palms facing down. The band should be taut with no slack. If you are using tube bands, you most likely won't use the handles.
2. Keeping arms straight, raise hands up to shoulder height in front of you with palms continuing to face down toward the floor.
3. Inhale then pull the band as your hands move outward and away from each other. Exhale as your hands is at the farthest point apart and your shoulder blades are squeezed. Inhale as you return your hands to the starting position. This is one rep.
4. Do 10 reps for 2 sets.

Make this more challenging by moving more slowly as you pull apart, then hold your hands apart and count to five. Slowly bring them back to the starting position.

Take Care:
There is a tendency for people to hunch up their shoulders while doing this exercise. Keep your shoulders down and neck loose.

SEE IT: youtu.be/-h-vQFYmYVM

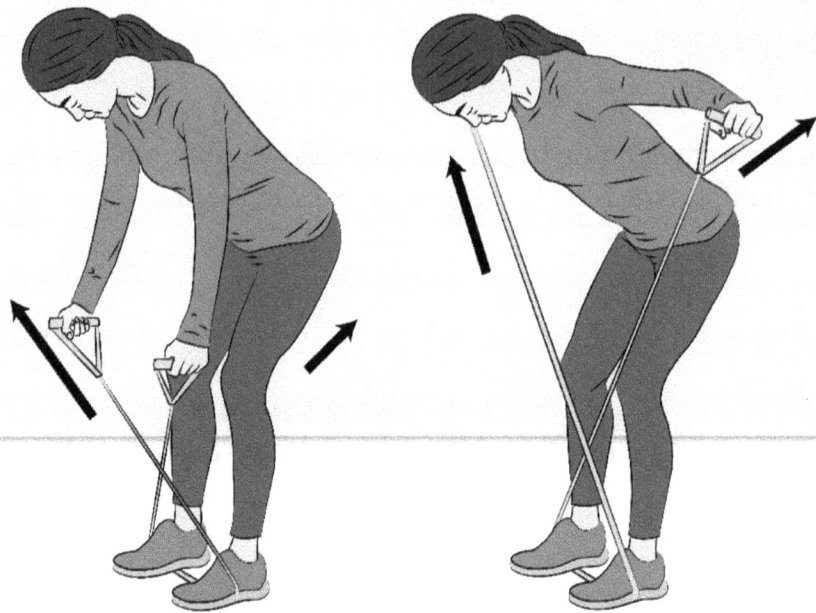

REVERSE FLY

BAND USED: THERAPY BAND OR A TUBE BAND WITH HANDLES | **TIME NEEDED:** 3 MINUTES

DIRECTIONS:

1. Stand with your feet hip-width distance apart. Step in the middle of the band and grab the handles in your hands. Hinge forward at the hip so that you are at a 45-degree angle with your arms out in front of you and fists toward the floor.
2. Inhale then bring your arms apart from each other on either side as you squeeze your shoulder blades together. Exhale as your arms is at the farthest point apart, then inhale as you bring your arms back to the starting position. This is one rep.
3. Do 10 reps for 2 sets.

Increase the difficulty by crisscrossing the band and grabbing the opposite handles so that it forms an "X" in front of you. This will increase the resistance.

Take Care:
Be aware of your back in this exercise. If hinging forward is difficult for you or causes you to lose your balance, do one arm at a time while placing the other hand on a countertop or sturdy chair for support.

SEE IT: healthline.com/health/fitness/back-exercises-with-bands

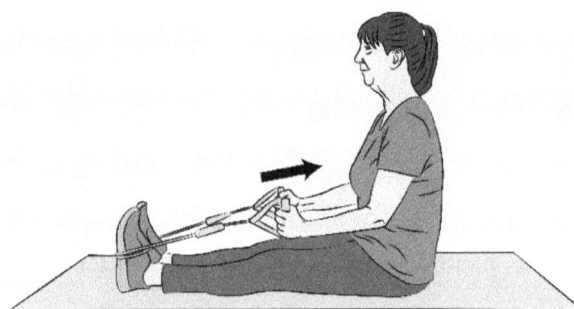

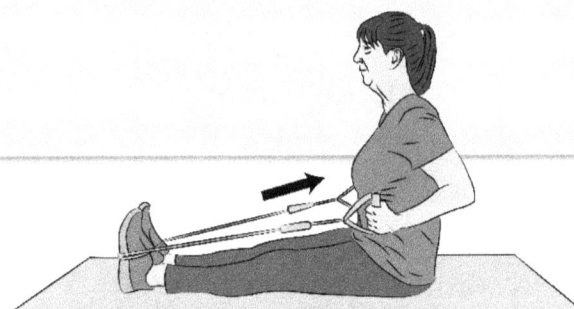

SEATED ROW

BAND USED: THERAPY BAND OR A TUBE BAND WITH HANDLES | **TIME NEEDED:** 3 MINUTES

DIRECTIONS:

1. Sit on the floor with legs together and feet extended straight out in front of you. Loop the middle of the band under the midsole area of your shoes.
2. Hold a handle in each hand with your palms facing each other. With arms extended in front of you, the band should not have any slack. If the band is too long, loop it around your feet to shorten it so the band is taut.

3. With your back erect and arms extended, inhale and bend your elbows as you draw your hands to your abdomen. Exhale as your elbows go back behind you and your shoulder blades squeeze together.
4. Inhale as your hands and arms return to the starting position. This is one rep.
5. Do 10 reps for 2 sets.

LEVEL UP:

To increase the difficulty, loop the band around your feet a couple of times to increase the resistance. Or you can switch to a thicker band.

Take Care:
Sit up tall and do not slouch as your arms extend.
The only thing moving in this exercise is your arms.
Don't bend forward.

SEE IT: youtu.be/6bvCuSeXLwc

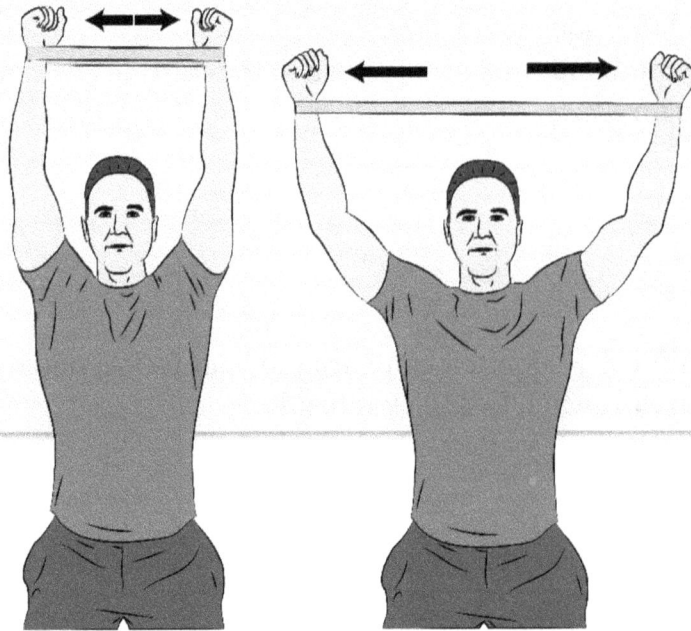

STANDING Y

BAND USED: MINI BAND | **TIME NEEDED:** 3 MINUTES

DIRECTIONS:

1. Stand up tall with feet hip-width distance apart. Place both hands through the mini band so that the band is at wrist level. Raise both arms so that your hands are up overhead.
2. Inhale then slowly move your hands away from each other so that your arms form a "Y" and exhale at the furthest point. Inhale as you bring your arms back to the starting position. This is one rep.
3. Do 10 reps for 2 sets.

Use a thicker mini band to increase the resistance.

Take Care:
This exercise is harder than you think! Start off with
a thin band with a low resistance
to avoid injury

SEE IT: healthline.com/health/fitness/back-exercises-with-bands

Chapter 5
Core and Glutes

The number one area that I encourage my clients to strengthen is their core muscles!

These muscles are key to maintaining your health and independence as you grow older. Our core isn't just the abdominal muscles but includes all the muscles in our torso, both front and back. They help you stand up, sit down, bend over, lift items, and accomplish daily tasks. The core muscles are absolutely needed for balance and body stability as you go about your day. The glutes are one area of the core that is especially important because of the heavy lifting they do in keeping our backs strong and protected.

Don't skip this chapter!

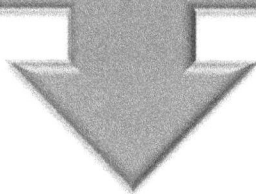

DON'T MISS THE CORE EXERCISES

Core

Exercises

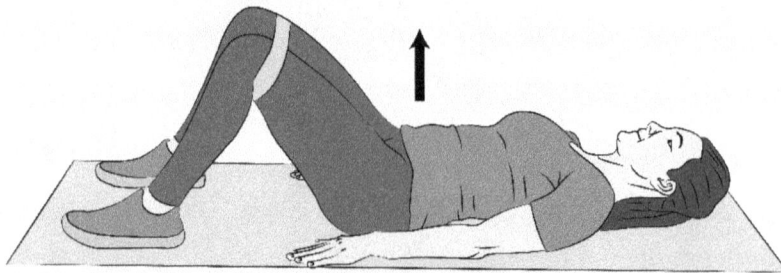

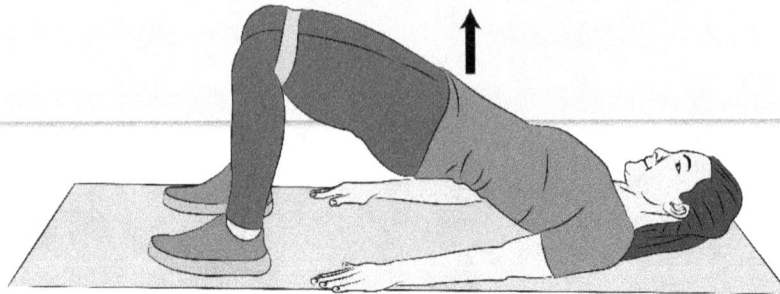

BRIDGE

BAND USED: MINI BAND | **TIME NEEDED:** 3 MINUTES

DIRECTIONS:

1. Sit down on the floor or on an exercise mat. Place both feet through a mini band and bring the band up to your thighs, just above your knees. Lie down on your back with your knees bent and both feet flat on the floor hip-width distance apart.
2. Inhale then raise your hips while pressing your upper back and heels into the floor. Exhale as your hips reach the top, then inhale as you return to the starting position. This is one rep.
3. Do 10 reps for 2 sets.

To increase the difficulty, hold for five seconds when your hips are raised before slowly lowering back down.

Take Care:
Watch that your knees do not flop outwards as you lift your hips.
Keep them parallel to each
other.

SEE IT: healthline.com/health/fitness/resistance-band-workouts-abs

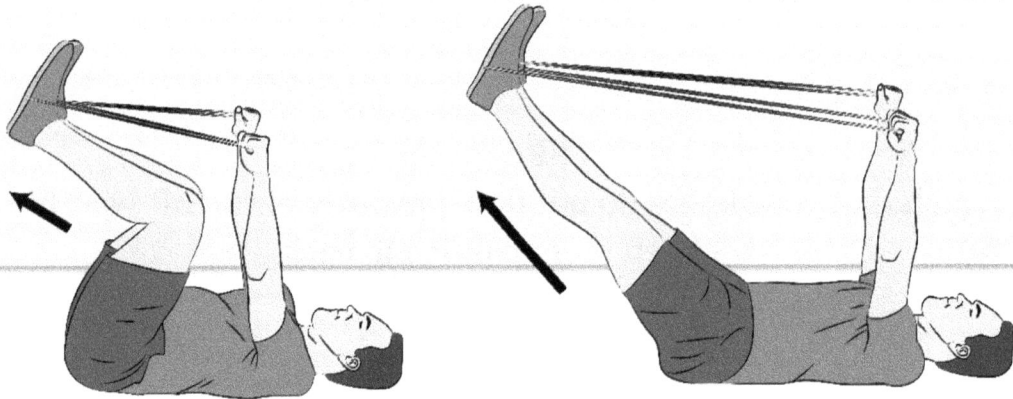

DOUBLE LEG STRETCH

BAND USED: LOOP BAND, THERAPY BAND, OR TUBE BAND WITH HANDLES
TIME NEEDED: 3 MINUTES

1. Sit down on the floor or exercise mat. Place the middle of the band under the bottom of your feet and grab the band ends in your hands. Lie down on your back and bring your knees up toward the ceiling and feet parallel to the floor. Your knees should be bent at a 90-degree angle.
2. Inhale and tighten your abs as you raise both hands toward the ceiling. Exhale as you extend both feet and straighten your legs so that they are at a 45-degree angle. Inhale as you return your legs to the starting position. This is one rep.
3. Do 10 reps for 2 sets.

To make this more challenging, when straightening your legs, bring them down to where they are just hovering above the floor before returning to the starting position. This is an advanced move!

Take Care
Don't lift your head or neck off the floor to avoid straining them.

SEE IT: healthline.com/health/fitness/resistance-band-workouts-abs

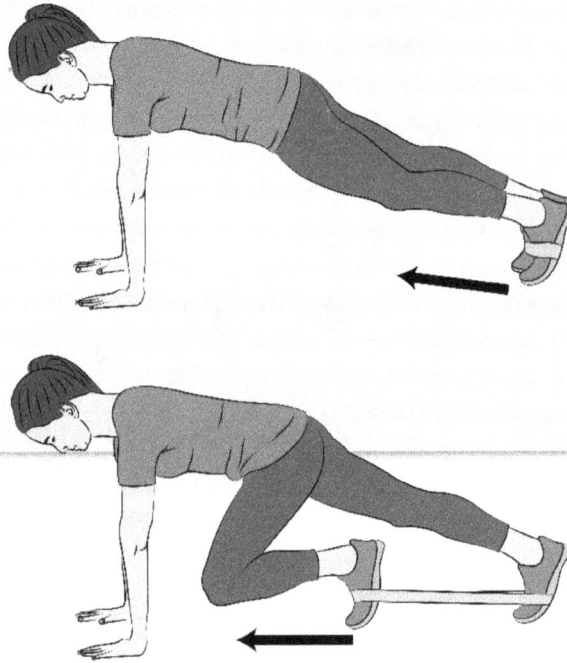

MOUNTAIN CLIMBER

BAND USED: MINI BAND | **TIME NEEDED:** 4 MINUTES

1. Place a mini band around both feet so that it is directly under both arches. Get into a straight-arm plank position facing down toward the floor and core engaged.
2. Inhale as you lift your right foot and bring your right knee up toward your right elbow. Exhale as it gets closer to your elbow, then inhale and bring your leg back to the starting position. Now, do the same with your left leg. This is one rep.
3. Do 10 reps for 2 sets.

To make this more difficult, you can either add speed by doing the move quicker or use a thicker band for more resistance.

Take Care
Don't allow your midsection and lower back to sag.
Keep your core tight throughout the
exercise.

SEE IT: healthline.com/health/fitness/resistance-band-workouts-abs

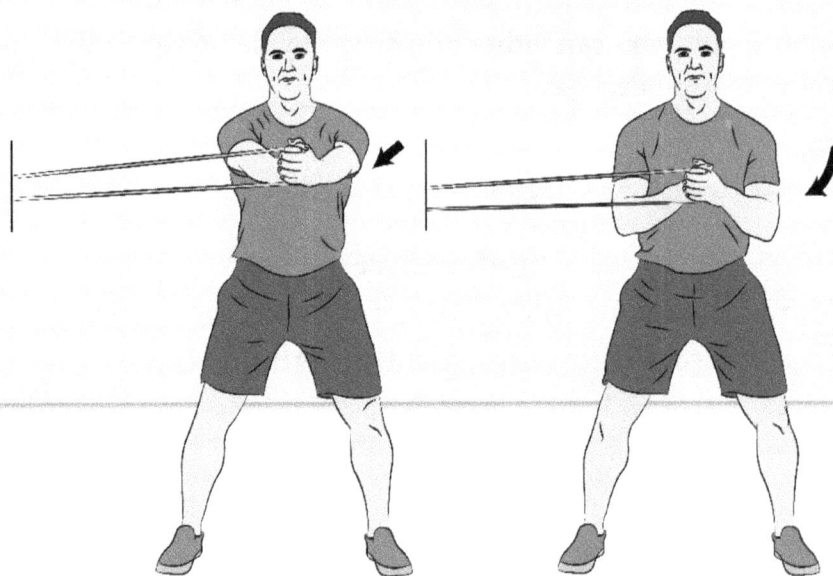

PALLOF PRESS

BAND USED: LONG LOOP BAND OR TUBE BAND WITH HANDLES | **TIME NEEDED:** 3 MINUTES

DIRECTIONS:

1. Anchor the band at chest height to a sturdy object or anchor point. Grab the other end of the loop with both hands. You can either interlace your fingers or have one hand over the other.
2. Turn your body so that the anchor point is directly to your right and there is no slack in the band. If you are kneeling or standing, your legs should be hip-width apart. If you are sitting, your feet should be flat on the floor.
3. Bend your arms at the elbow and hold your hands at the front of your chest. Inhale as extend your hands straight out in front of you, keeping them at chest height and

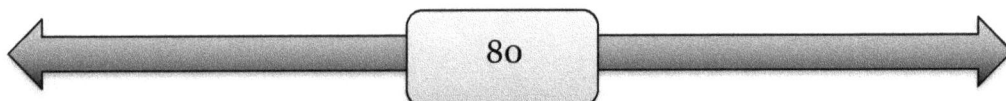

engaging your core. Keep your torso taut and don't allow it to twist. Exhale as your hands reach the farthest point, then inhale as you bring them back to the starting position. This is one rep.

4. Do 10 reps for 2 sets.

LEVEL UP:

To make this more difficult, you can change your stance to a standing staggered position or a squat position. This will challenge your balance as well.

Take Care
This can be done standing, seated, or kneeling.
Be sure to adjust the anchor point so that it is at chest height
Whatever position you are in.

SEE IT: livestrong.com/article/108869-resistance-band-exercises-seniors/

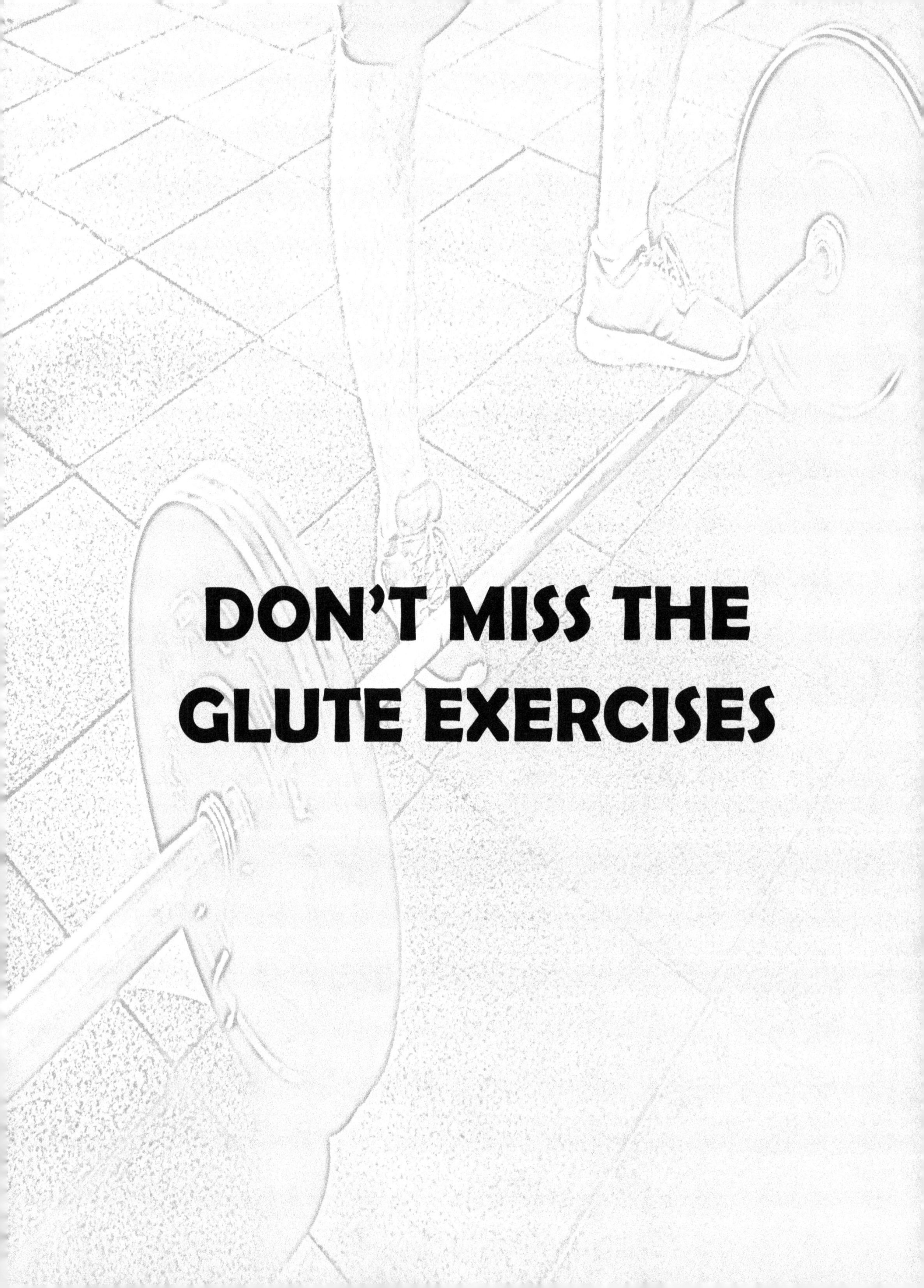

DON'T MISS THE GLUTE EXERCISES

Glute
Exercises

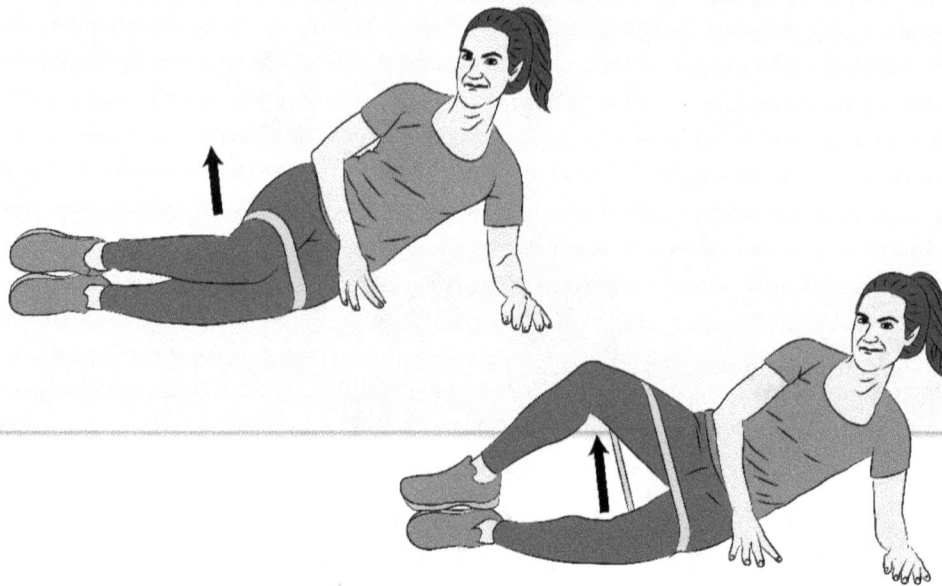

CLAM SHELL

BAND USED: MINI BAND OR THERAPY BAND | **TIME NEEDED:** 4 MINUTES

DIRECTIONS:

1. Sit down on the floor or on an exercise mat. Place both feet through a mini band or tie a therapy band around your thighs. Bring the band onto your thighs just above your knees.
2. Lie down on your right side and bend your knees at a 90-degree angle. Your hips, knees, and ankles should be stacked on top of each other. Prop up your upper body onto your right elbow and forearm for support.

3. Keep your feet together as you inhale and raise your left knee up toward the sky. Exhale at the top and inhale as you bring your knee back down to the starting position. This is one rep.
4. Do 10 reps for 2 sets on this side. Switch to the other side and lie on your left side. This time, raise your right knee for 10 reps and 2 sets.

To make this more of a challenge, hold your knee at the top of the move for 5 seconds before lowering back down.

Take Care
Keep your core and back engaged so that you don't allow your torso to roll toward the front or back as you do the exercise.

SEE IT: self.com/gallery/5-effective-resistance-band-exercises-for-a-strong-firm-butt

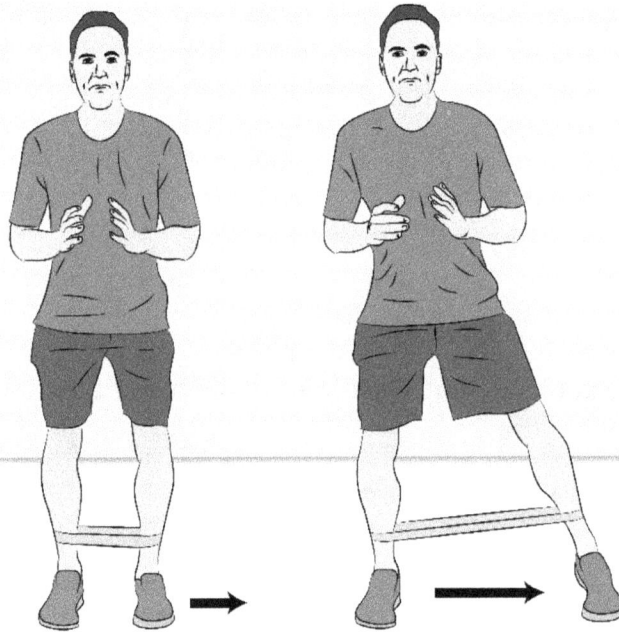

SCISSOR TOE TAP

BAND USED: MINI BAND | **TIME NEEDED:** 4 MINUTES

DIRECTIONS:

1. Step both feet through a mini band. Bring the band up so it is around your ankles. Stand with your feet hip-width distance apart and your hands on your hips. There should be no slack in your band.

2. Take a step back with your right foot to a 45-degree angle. If you were standing in the middle of a clockface, your right toes would be tapping back into the 5 o'clock position. Don't twist your torso and keep your hips pointing straight ahead. Bring your foot back to the starting position. This is one rep.

3. Do 10 reps for 2 sets with your right foot. Switch and do the same with your left foot.

Make this more challenging by holding your toes out when they tap back for a few seconds before returning to the starting position.

Take Care:
If you need extra balance support, place one or both hands on a Sturdy chair or countertop while performing this exercise.

SEE IT: livestrong.com/article/108869-resistance-band-exercises-seniors/

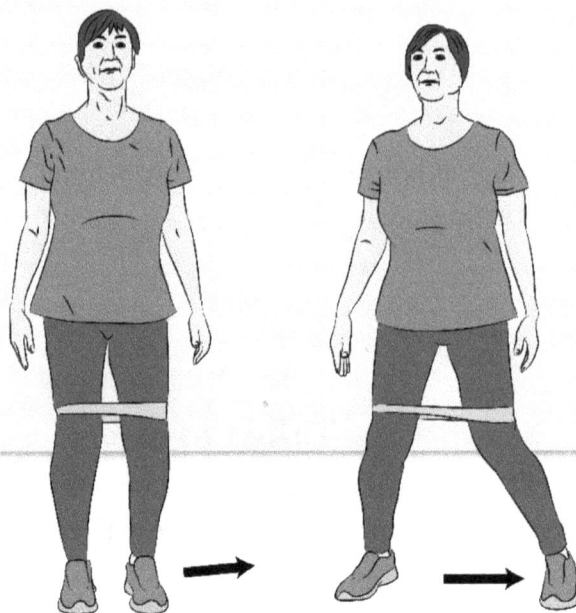

SIDE STEP

BAND USED: MINI BAND | **TIME NEEDED:** 4 MINUTES

DIRECTIONS:

1. Place both feet through a mini band. Bring the band up to your thighs just above your knees. Stand with your feet hip-width distance apart and bend your knees slightly.
2. Breathe normally as you step your right foot to the right six inches and follow with your left foot following it. Continue to step to the right five times in total. Now, go in the opposite direction and step to your left five times. This is one rep.
3. Do 5 reps for 2 sets.

Challenge yourself by either moving the band down to your ankles and performing the exercise or adding an additional band at your ankles.

Take Care
Keep your core engaged as you perform this lateral move.
It will help you keep your balance.

SEE IT: youtu.be/u7Rylyi1Zwg

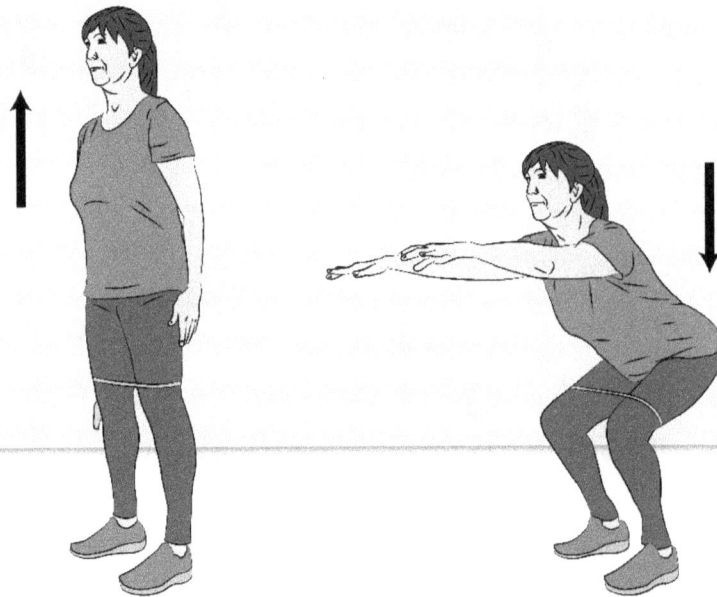

SQUATS

BAND USED: MINI BAND | **TIME NEEDED:** 3 MINUTES

DIRECTIONS:

1. Step both feet through a mini band. Bring the band up to your thighs just above your knees. Place feet hip-width distance apart.
2. Inhale as you bend your knees and lower your buttocks as if you were going to sit down in a chair. Lower down only as far as comfortable and that you are able to keep your balance. Exhale as you stand up and return to the starting position. This is one rep.
3. Do 10 reps for 2 or 3 sets.

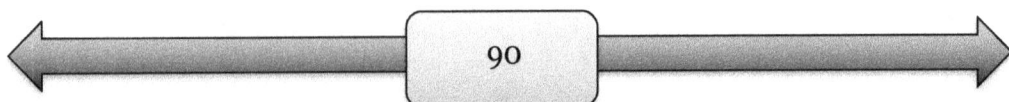

To increase the difficulty, use a thicker band for more resistance or lower your buttocks lower.

Take Care:
Watch your balance while doing this exercise.
If needed, hold on to a countertop or sturdy chair to avoid falling.

SEE IT: youtu.be/fgAOisQy_sI

Chapter 6
Quads and Hamstrings

Your quadriceps muscles, or quads, and hamstrings are the principal muscles in your thighs. They support your legs, torso, and body throughout the day and allow you to stand, sit, walk, and run. Strengthening these muscles makes sense to not only keep your mobility and balance, but these muscles are also important to preventing knee pain and decreasing your risk for injury. The quads are the muscles on the front of your thighs while the hamstrings run along the back of your thighs from the glutes down toward your knees. They work in association with each other, much like the biceps and triceps in your arm do.

Don't skip the Quad Exercises!

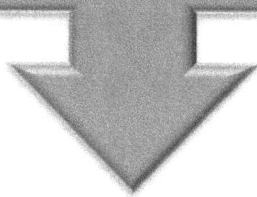

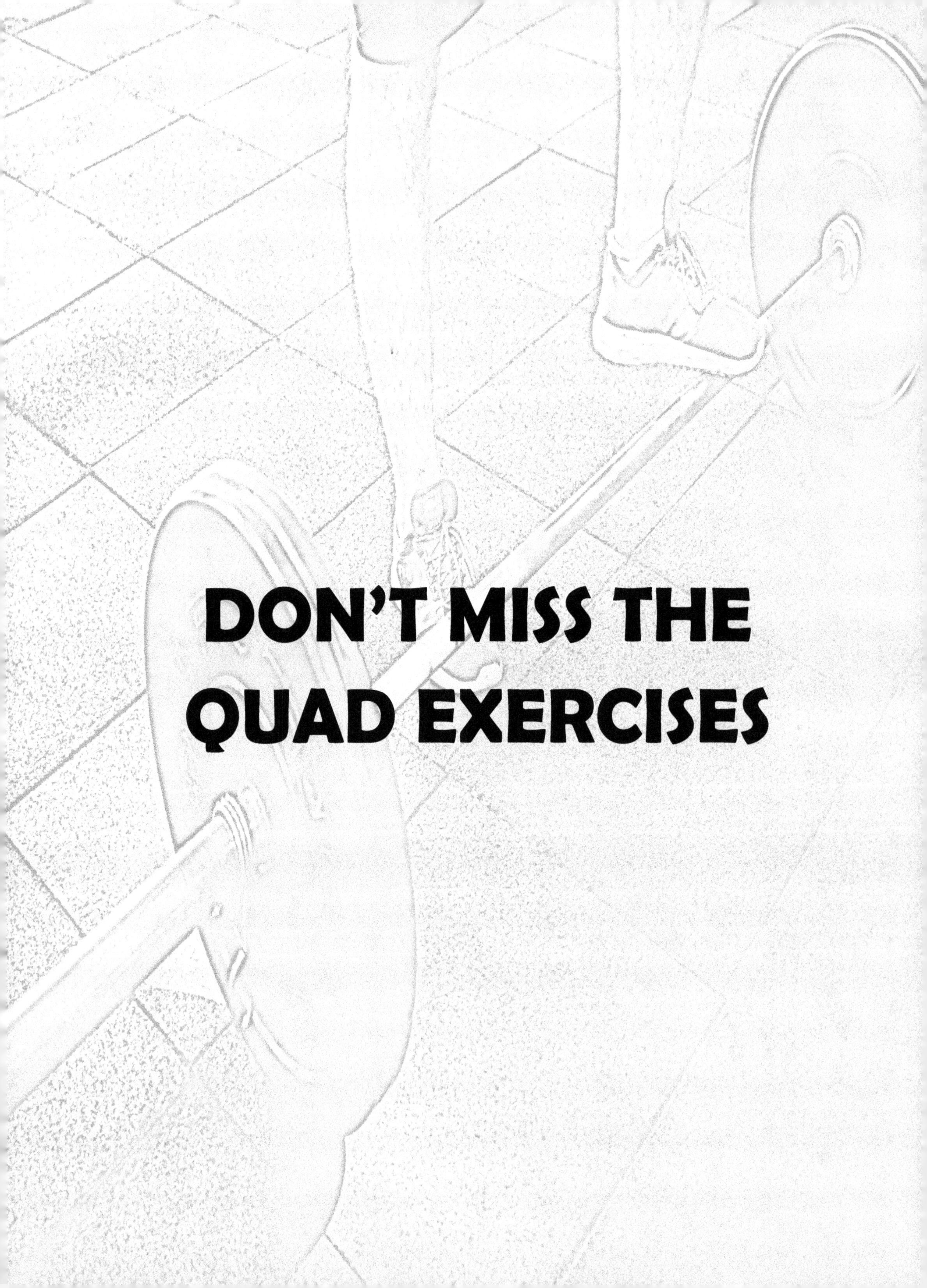

DON'T MISS THE QUAD EXERCISES

Quad Exercises

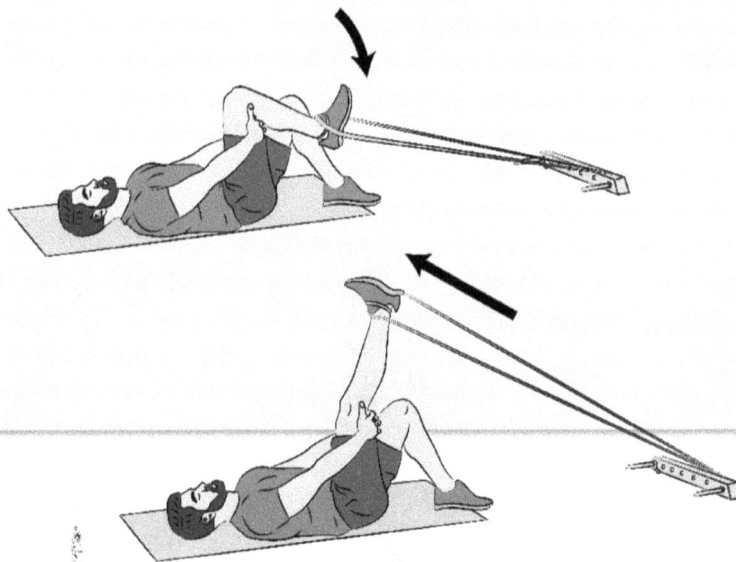

BANDED LEG EXTENSION

BAND USED: LOOP BAND OR TUBE BAND WITH HANDLES |
TIME NEEDED: 4 MINUTES

DIRECTIONS:

1. Anchor one end of the band to an anchor point or sturdy object at floor level. Lie down on the floor or on an exercise mat facing up and with your feet pointing toward the anchor point. Loop the free end of the band around your right ankle. Bend both knees and place your feet flat on the floor.

2. Raise your right knee and place your hands around the back of your right thigh, holding on to it. Inhale as you straighten your right leg and lift your right foot toward the sky. Exhale at the top as you squeeze your right quad muscle, then inhale as you lower your foot back to the starting position. This is one rep.

3. Do 10 reps for 2 sets on this side. Switch sides and repeat on the left.

As you get stronger, see if you can do this exercise without holding on to your thigh.

Take Care
Keep your lower back pressed to the floor and don't
allow it to arch.

SEE IT: thefitnessphantom.com/resistance-band-quad-exercises

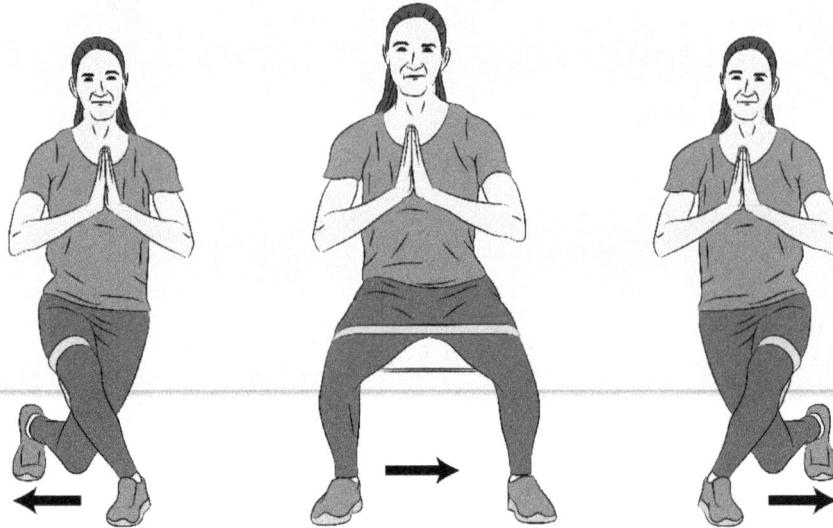

CURTSY SQUAT

BAND USED: MINI BAND OR THERAPY BAND | **TIME NEEDED:** 4 MINUTES

DIRECTIONS:

1. Step both feet through a mini band or tie a therapy band around your thighs. Bring the band up to your thighs just above the knees. Stand with feet hip-width distance apart.
2. Bend both knees as if you were going to do a squat, then bring your right foot and right knee behind your left knee to do a curtsy. Only squat down as far as comfortable while keeping your balance. Stand back up and bring your right foot back to the starting position. This is one rep.

3. Do 10 reps for 2 sets. Switch to the other foot and repeat.

As you get stronger, alternate sides each time you perform the curtsy squats rather than just sticking to one side.

Take Care
This is a balance-challenging exercise as well, so take care to stabilize yourself if needed by having one hand on a countertop or sturdy chair.

SEE IT: thefitnessphantom.com/resistance-band-quad-exercises

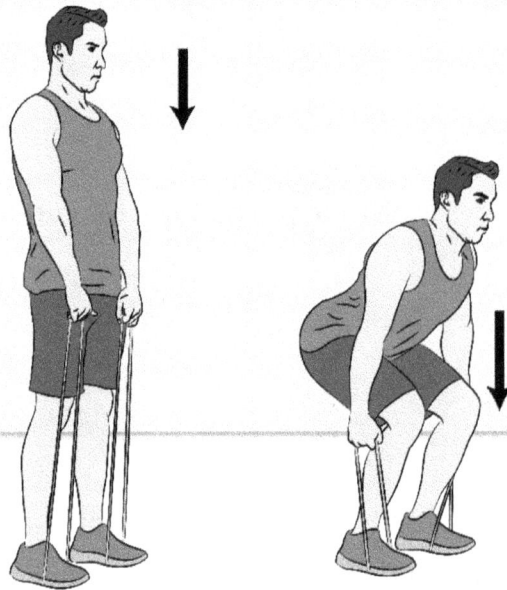

DEADLIFT

BAND USED: LOOP BAND OR TUBE BAND WITH HANDLES | **TIME NEEDED:** 3 MINUTES

DIRECTIONS:

1. Stand with feet hip-width distance apart. Place the center of the band under both feet. Grab the ends with either hand. Start in a squat position, hinged at the hips and back flat. The band should be taut with no slack.
2. Inhale then slowly exhale as you stand up straight, pulling on the bands. Inhale as you return to the starting position. This is one rep.
3. Do 10 reps for 2 sets.

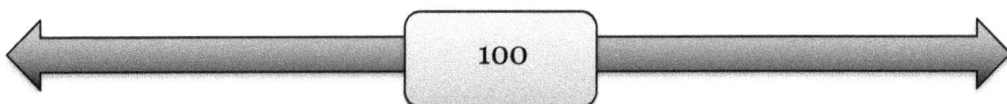

Make this more difficult by using a thicker band or by using more than one loop band at a time.

Take Care
Pay attention to your back and don't allow it to hunch forward.
Keep your spine straight as you stand up.

SEE IT: thefitnessphantom.com/resistance-band-quad-exercises

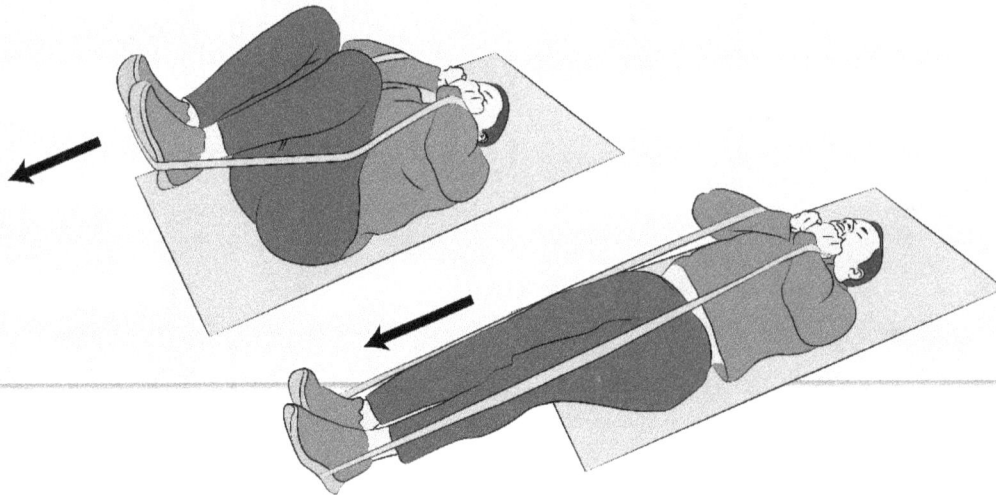

LYING LEG PRESS

BAND USED: LARGE LOOP BAND OR TUBE BAND WITH HANDLES | **TIME NEEDED:** 3 MINUTES

DIRECTIONS:

1. Lie down on the floor or on an exercise mat. Bend your knees and bring them up toward your chest. Place one end of the loop band under the arches of both feet. If using a tube band, place the middle of the band under your feet. Grab the other end of the band with both hands. Bend your arms and place your hands on your chest.
2. Inhale then exhale as you press down on the band and straighten your legs. Inhale as you bend your legs and return them to the starting position. This is one rep.
3. Do 10 reps for 3 sets.

Increase the intensity by choosing a thicker band with more resistance.

Take Care
Don't allow your neck or back to rise up off the floor.
Keep them resting on the floor and your
back straight.

SEE IT: thefitnessphantom.com/resistance-band-quad-exercises

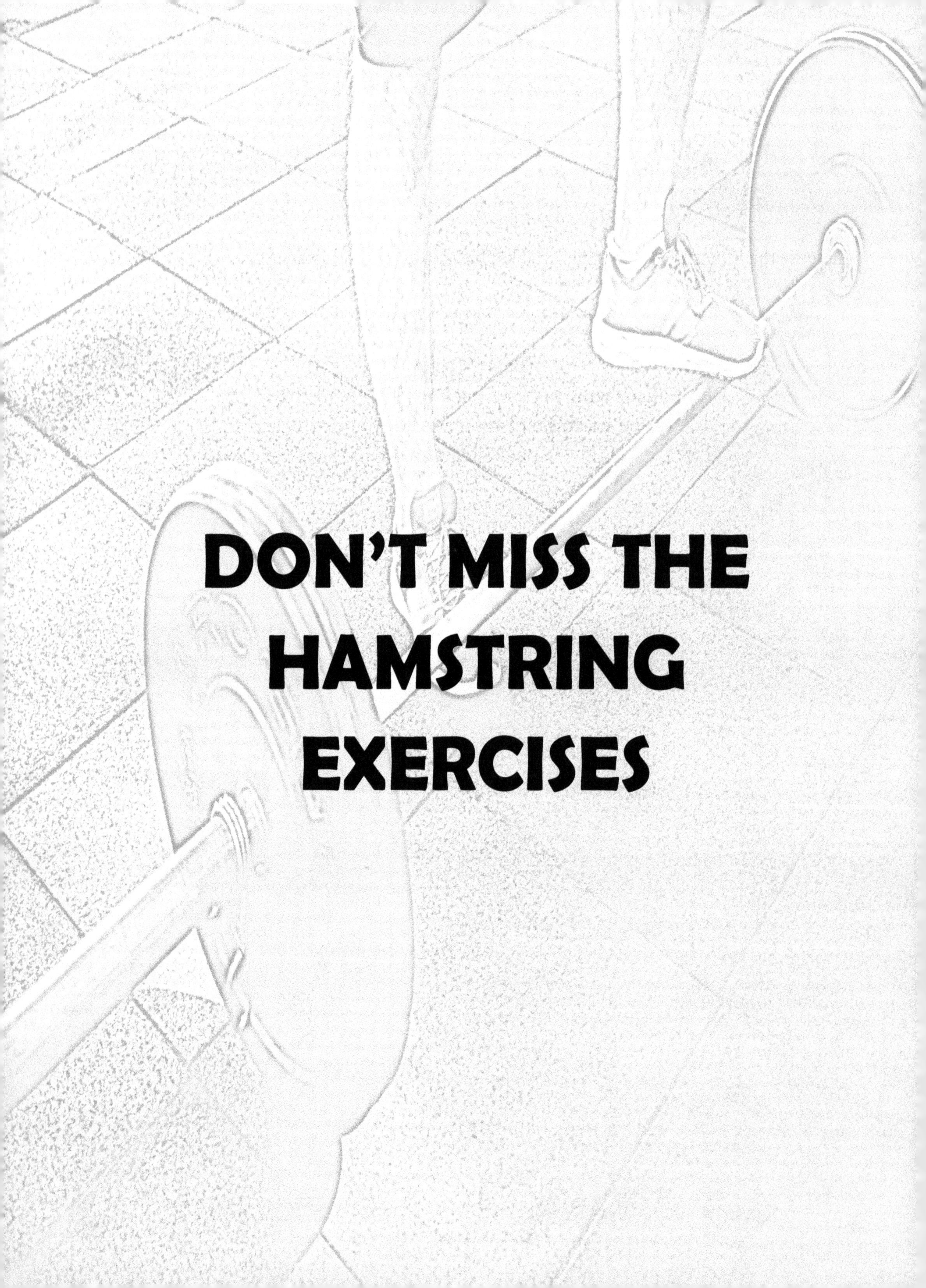

DON’T MISS THE HAMSTRING EXERCISES

Hamstring

Exercises

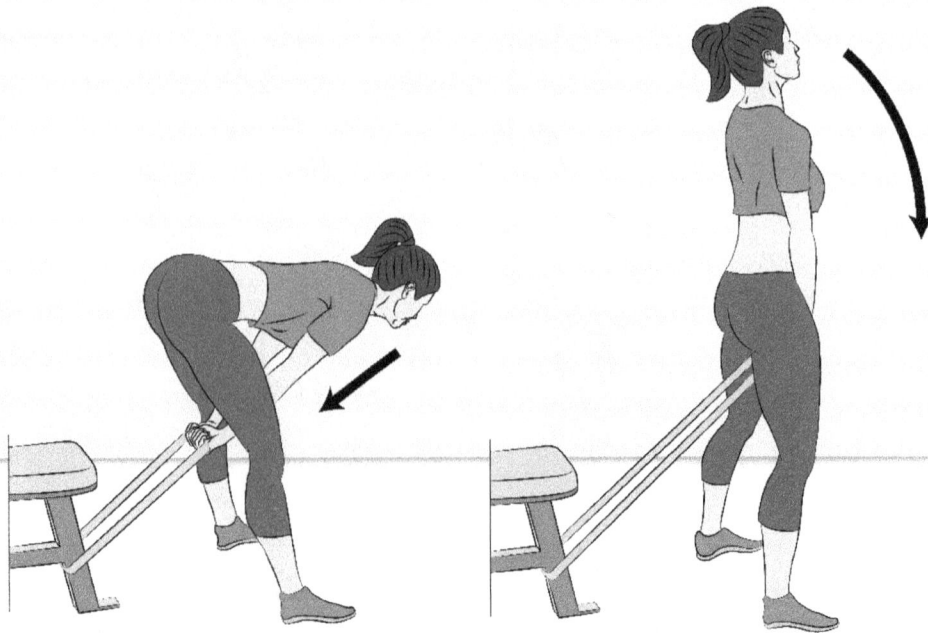

BAND PULL THROUGH

BAND USED: LOOP BAND, THERAPY BAND, OR TUBE BAND WITH HANDLES |
TIME NEEDED: 3 MINUTES

DIRECTIONS:

1. Anchor one end of the band to an anchor point down near the floor. Walk far enough away from the anchor point so that the band is taut. Face away from the anchor point and grab the other end of the band so that it is between your legs.
2. Stand with your feet shoulder-width apart and hinge forward at the hips. Keeping your arms straight and holding on to the band, inhale and stand up straight. You should feel your hamstrings working as you stand. If not, take one step away to make

the band tighter. Exhale at the top, then inhale as you hinge forward and return to the starting position. This is one rep.

3. Do 10 reps for 3 sets.

LEVEL UP:

You can make this harder by taking another step away from the anchor point or switching to a thicker band.

Take Care
Don't let momentum take over here! It's easy to start swinging your hips forward but keep your movements slow and controlled and squeeze your glutes when you stand up.

SEE IT: coachsofiafitness.com/5-resistance-band-hamstrings-exercises

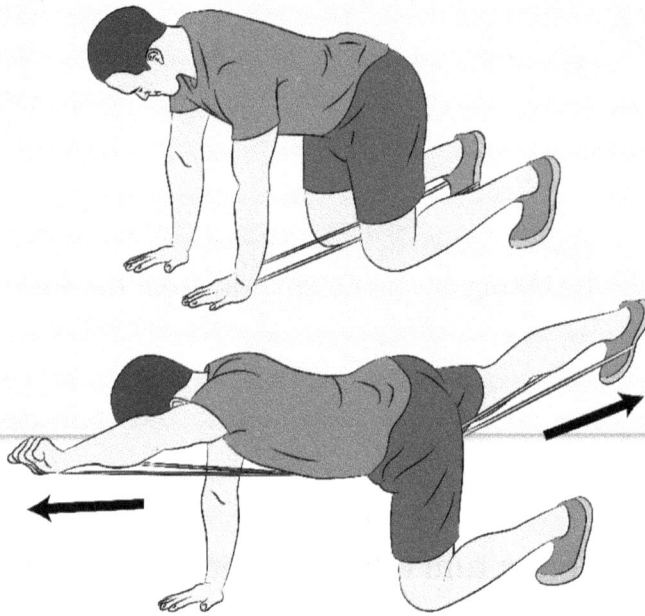

BIRD DOG

BAND USED: LOOP BAND OR TUBE BAND WITH HANDLES | **TIME NEEDED:** 4 MINUTES

DIRECTIONS:

1. Get down on the floor or exercise mat on your hands and knees. Loop one end of the band under the arch of your right foot and grab the other end of the band with the opposite (the left) hand.
2. Inhale and tighten your core as you lift your left hand and right foot at the same time and extend them out straight, so they are parallel to the floor. Exhale as they are fully extended, then inhale and return them to the starting position. This is one rep.

3. Do 10 reps and 2 sets with this hand and foot. Switch to the opposite hand and foot and repeat.

LEVEL UP:

Challenge yourself by holding for five seconds while your arm and leg are fully extended before returning to the starting position.

Take Care
Be mindful of your back while doing this exercise.
Don't arch your back, but keep it long and neutral. If you find this exercise too difficult, start off with both hands on the floor and just move your legs.

SEE IT: healthline.com/health/fitness/resistance-band-workouts-abs

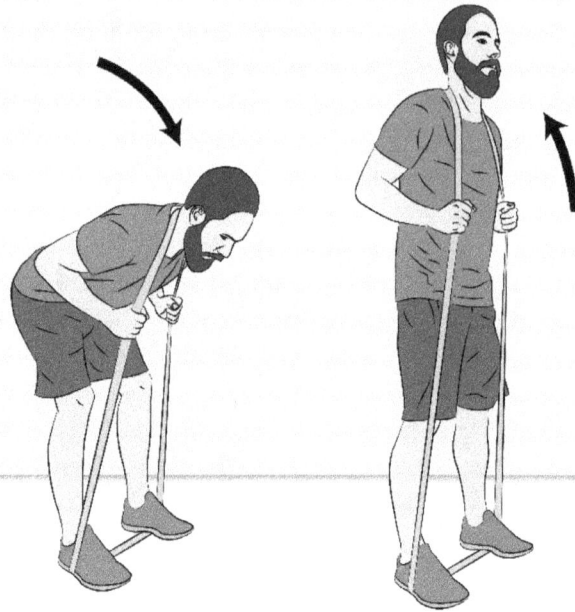

GOOD MORNINGS

BAND USED: LONG LOOP BAND | **TIME NEEDED:** 3 MINUTES

DIRECTIONS:

1. Stand with your feet hip-width distance apart. Loop one end of the band under your feet and stand on it firmly. Hinge forward at the hips and loop the other end of the band over your head and around the back of your neck or upper shoulders.
2. Keep a slight bend in your knees and your backs straight as you bend forward until nearly parallel to the floor. Inhale, then exhale as you raise up to a standing position. Inhale as you return to the starting position. This is one rep.
3. Do 10 reps for 3 sets.

Make this move more difficult by moving very slowly through the exercise and really squeezing your hamstrings and glutes as you stand.

Take Care:
Watch that your neck doesn't bend forward
or become irritated by the band. Place a small towel or cloth to prevent chafing. If you have had neck surgery or have neck issues, avoid the neck by placing the band across your upper shoulder and holding on to it with your hands.

SEE IT: thefitnessphantom.com/resistance-band-hamstring-exercises

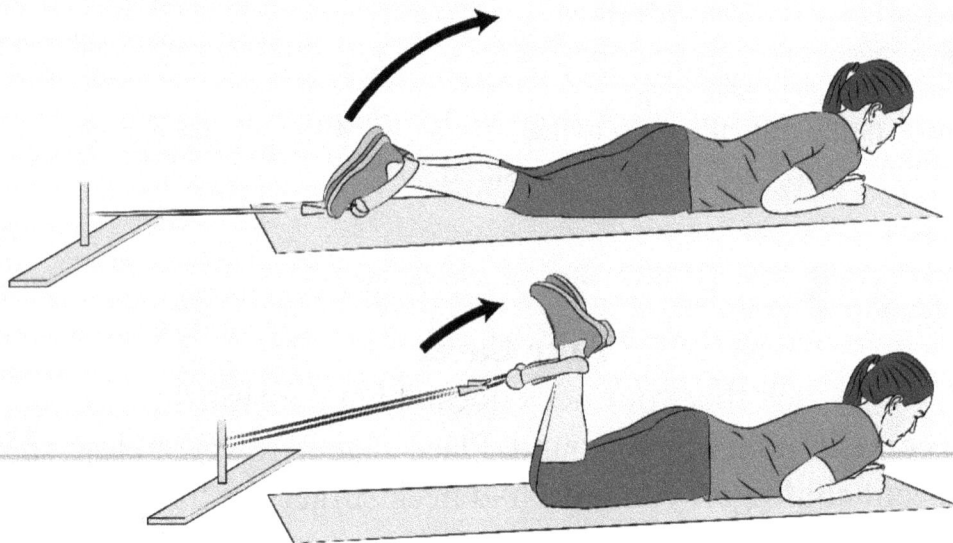

LYING LEG CURL

BAND USED: LOOP BAND OR TUBE BAND WITH HANDLES | **TIME NEEDED:** 3 MINUTES

DIRECTIONS:

1. Anchor one end of the band at an anchor point near the floor. Loop the other end of the band onto your ankles. Lie down face down on your stomach on the floor or on an exercise mat. Your feet should be pointing toward the anchor point.

2. Inhale then bend your knees and bring your feet up toward your buttocks. Exhale as your feet get closer to your butt. Inhale as you lower your feet and straighten your legs back to the starting position. This is one rep.

3. Do 10 reps for 3 sets.

To increase the resistance and make this more difficult, scootch yourself a little farther away from the anchor point or use a thicker band.

Take Care:
You can prop your upper body up on your forearms or lie down, resting your forehead on your hands, whichever is more comfortable for your back.

SEE IT: thefitnessphantom.com/resistance-band-hamstring-exercises

Chapter 7
Forearms and Calves

W hile we don't think too much about the smaller muscles in our forearms and calves, think about how much they do for us! The muscles in our forearms are many times some of the weakest because they are often overlooked in strength training. Our forearms are the gateway muscles to overall arm strength. Our biceps and triceps need strong forearms to effectively do their jobs. Forearm muscles also are essential for grip strength to help us accomplish tasks like opening jars and performing fine motor skills with the hands and wrists. Calves play a similar role in our legs. We need strong calf muscles for our legs to function properly. Our calves help to support ankle mobility and stability, which is essential in standing, walking, and stepping over objects. These muscles also contribute to our feet and heels as they support our body and posture.

Let's work these muscles

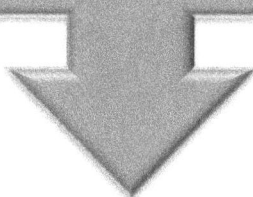

DON'T MISS THE FOREARMS EXERCISES

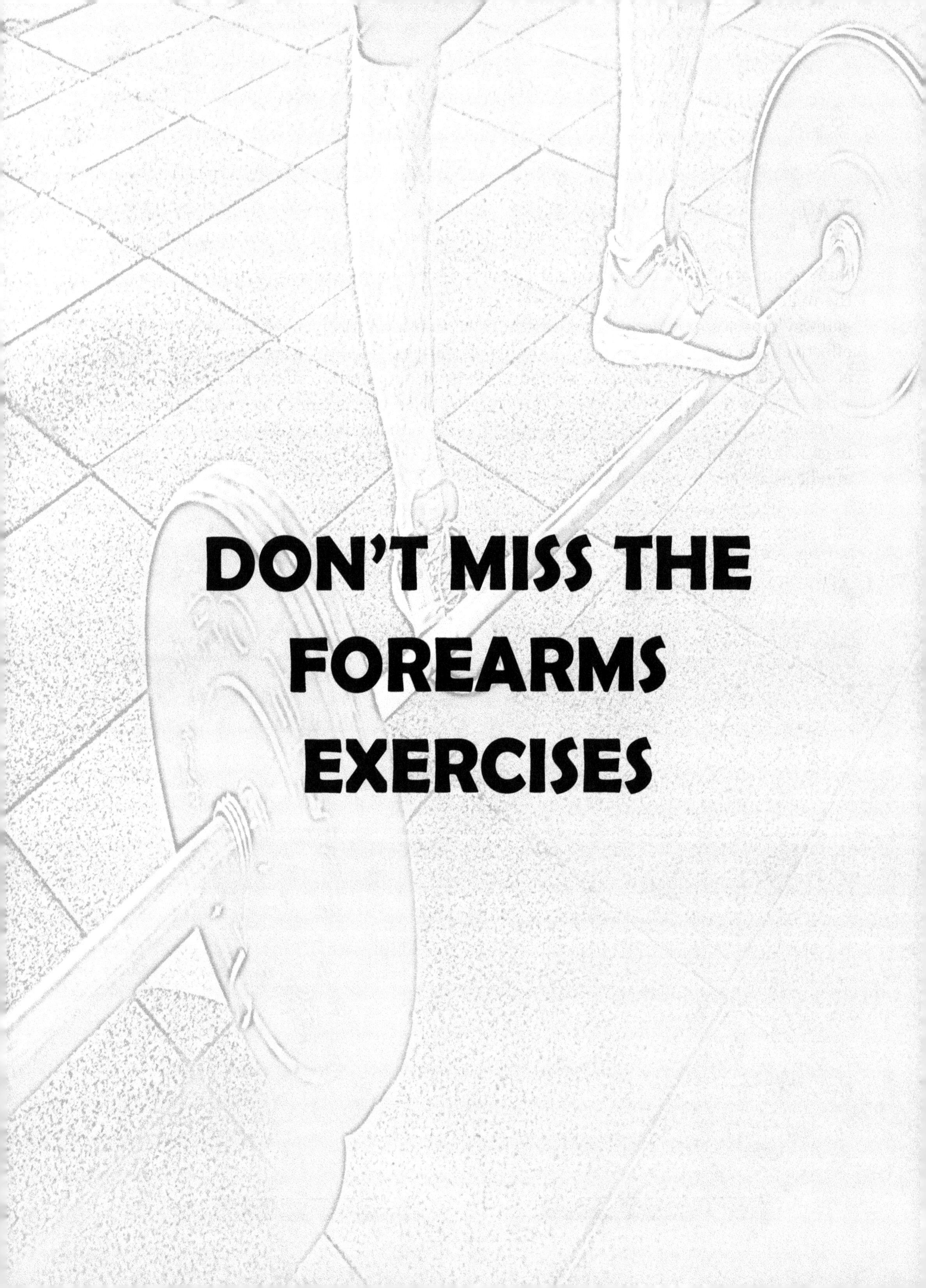

Forearms

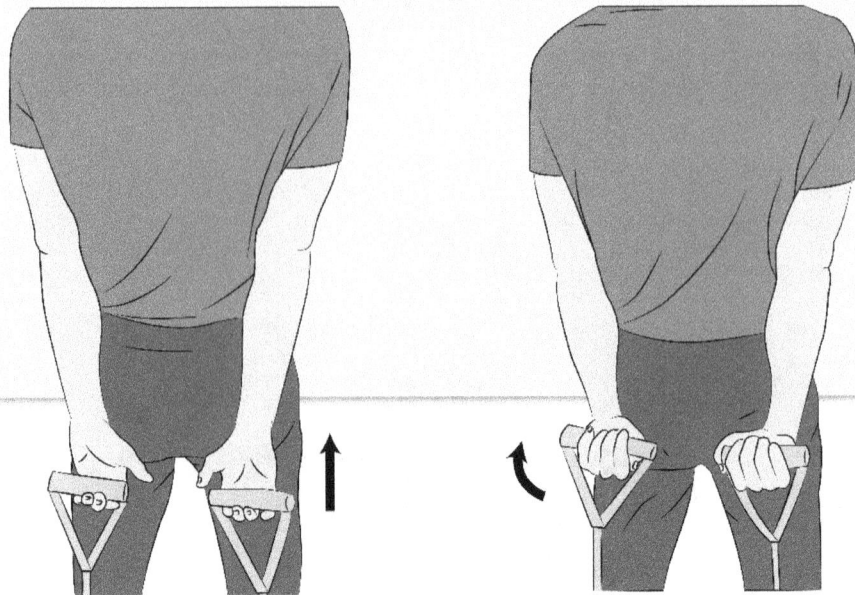

BEHIND THE BACK WRIST CURL

BAND USED: THERAPY BAND OR TUBE BAND WITH HANDLES | **TIME NEEDED:** 3 MINUTES

DIRECTIONS:

1. Step on the middle of the band with both feet and stand with feet a hip-width distance apart. Grab the band ends or handles in your hands. Bring your hands behind you so that the back of your hands is resting on your buttocks and your palms are facing out.
2. Inhale as you bend your wrists. Curl fists up away from your buttocks and toward your forearms, exhaling as you reach the top. Inhale as you slowly lower your hands back to the starting position. This is one rep.

3. Do 15 reps for 3 sets.

Challenge yourself by holding the curl for five seconds before lowering back to the starting position.

Take Care
Pay attention to your posture while doing this exercise.
Don't allow your shoulders to hunch up and
keep your arms as straight as possible.

SEE IT: criticalbody.com/resistance-band-forearm-exercises/

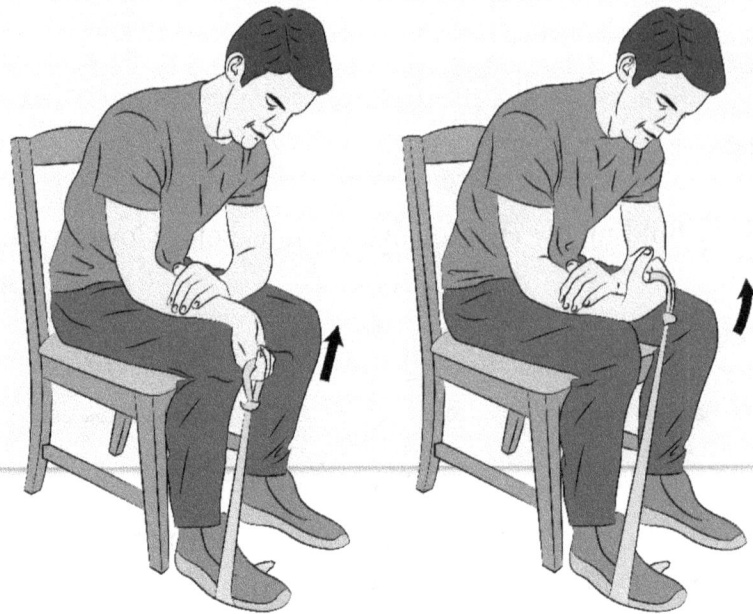

FOREARM CURL

BAND USED: LOOP BAND, THERAPY BAND, OR TUBE BAND WITH HANDLES | **TIME NEEDED:** 4 MINUTES

DIRECTIONS:

1. Sit down on a sturdy chair. Loop one end of the band under your right foot and hold the other end in your right hand. Allow your forearm to rest on the top of your right thigh with your palm facing up as you hold the band.
2. Inhale as you flex your forearm and curl your right wrist and hand up toward the inside of your right forearm. Exhale as your hand reaches the top of the move and then inhale as you return your hand to the starting position. This is one rep.
3. Do 15 reps for 3 sets on this arm. Switch to the left arm and repeat.

Add more sets to make this more difficult.

Take Care
Maintain good posture as you perform this exercise
and don't slump your shoulders forward.

SEE IT: criticalbody.com/resistance-band-forearm-exercises/

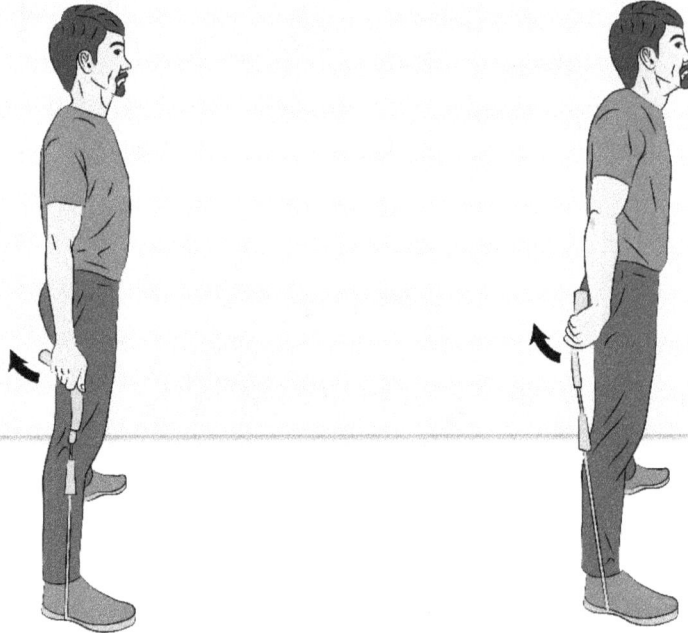

REAR ROTATION

BAND USED: THERAPY BAND | **TIME NEEDED:** 3 MINUTES

DIRECTIONS:

1. Stand in the middle of the band with your feet a hip-width distance apart. Grab the ends of the band with your hands and place your arms at your sides. Palms should face inward toward your body.
2. Keeping your arms straight, inhale and bend your wrists to the rear as you press your fists back. Exhale as you reach the maximum that your wrists can bend back, then inhale as they return to the starting point. This is one rep.
3. Do 15 reps for 3 sets.

This is a small move that works the underside of your forearms. Add more reps or sets to increase the difficulty.

Take Care
Use a lighter resistance band for this exercise
until your forearms get stronger.

SEE IT: criticalbody.com/resistance-band-forearm-exercises/

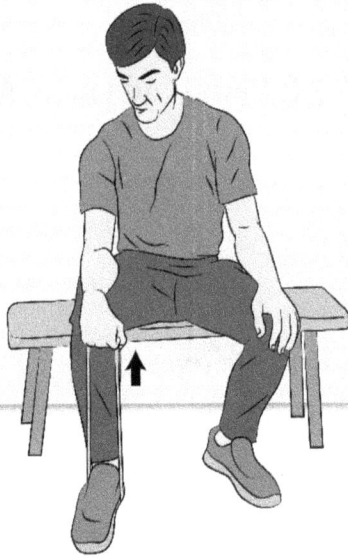

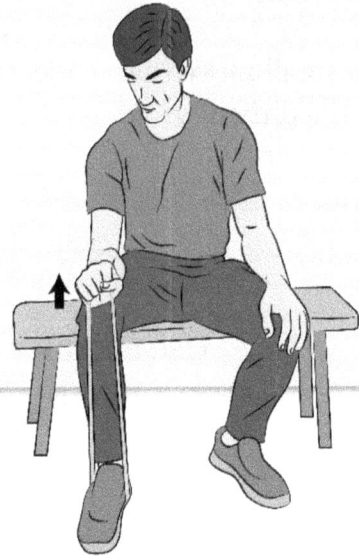

REVERSE FOREARM CURLS

BAND USED: LOOP BAND, THERAPY BAND, OR TUBE BAND WITH HANDLES | **TIME NEEDED:** 4 MINUTES

DIRECTIONS:

1. Sit down on a sturdy chair. Loop one end of the band under your right foot and hold the other end in your right hand. Allow your forearm to rest on the top of your right thigh with your palm facing down as you hold the band. This is very similar to the forearm curl, but with the palm facing down this time.
2. Inhale as you flex your forearm and curl your right wrist and hand up toward the sky. Exhale as your hand reaches the top of the move and then inhale as you return your hand to the starting position. This is one rep.
3. Do 15 reps for 3 sets on this arm. Switch to the left arm and repeat.

The move here is very small, so don't expect a big motion. Add more sets to make this more difficult.

Take Care

Maintain good posture as you perform this exercise.
If it helps you, rest your forearm on a table instead and allow your hand and wrist to come
out over the edge.

SEE IT: criticalbody.com/resistance-band-forearm-exercises/

DON'T MISS THE CALF EXERCISES

Calf Exercises

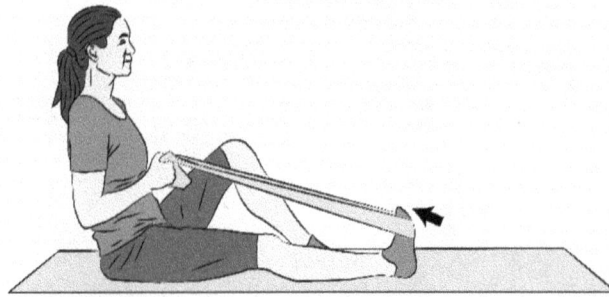

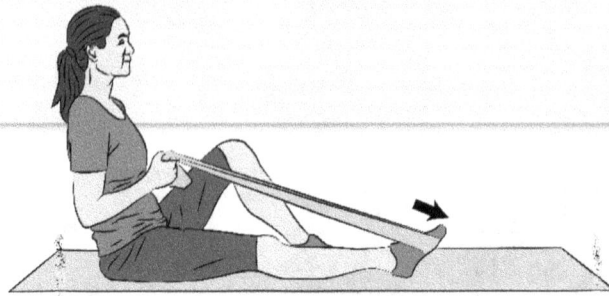

ANKLE PUMPS

BAND USED: LOOP BAND OR MINI BAND | **TIME NEEDED:** 4 MINUTES

1. Sit down on the floor or on an exercise mat. Loop one end of the band around your right foot under the arch and straighten your right leg. Grab the other end of the band with your left hand. Bend your left leg with your left foot flat on the floor.
2. Sit up tall with your right foot flexed and your toes pointed toward the sky. Inhale as you point your right toes away from you as if you were stepping on a gas pedal. Exhale when they are at the farthest point and inhale as you bring your foot back to the starting position. This is one rep.
3. Do 15 reps for 2 sets on this side. Switch legs and hands to do your left calf and repeat.

Not feeling the burn? Add reps or sets to increase the difficulty.

Take Care
Keep your back erect and don't slouch as you do this exercise.

SEE IT: livestrong.com/article/103743-resistance-band-calf-exercises

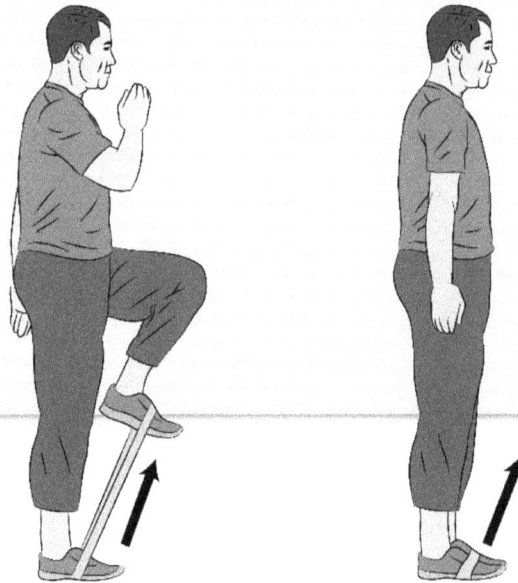

MARCHES WITH CALF RAISE

BAND USED: MINI BAND | **TIME NEEDED:** 3 MINUTES

DIRECTIONS:

1. Place a mini band around both feet so that the band is across the top of the feet and under the balls of the feet. Stand with feet a hip-width distance apart.
2. Inhale as you raise your right foot and bend your right knee, lifting it up toward the sky. At the same time, come up on the ball of your left foot and exhale. Inhale as you lower back down to the starting position. This is one rep.
3. Do 15 reps and 3 sets on this side. Switch legs and repeat on the left leg.

Increase the difficulty by alternating legs each time you raise your foot.

Take Care
This is also a challenge for your balance.
If you find yourself unsteady, place a hand on a
countertop or sturdy chair for extra stability.

SEE IT: livestrong.com/article/103743-resistance-band-calf-exercises

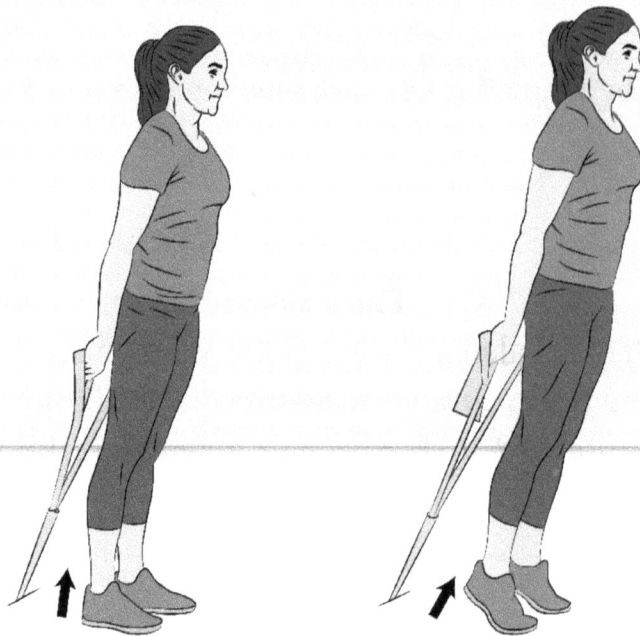

STANDING CALF RAISE WITH FLAT BAND

BAND USED: THERAPY BAND | **TIME NEEDED:** 3 MINUTES

1. Anchor the middle of the band to an anchor point at the bottom of a door or near the floor. Grab the ends of the band in each hand, facing away from the anchor point. Stand with your feet a hip-width distance apart and step forward until the band is taut.

2. Keep your arms straight and down by your sides or slightly behind your hips. Inhale as you raise up onto the balls of your feet. Exhale as you reach the top of the move, then inhale as you slowly lower your heels back down to the ground. This is one rep.
3. Do 15 reps for 3 sets.

LEVEL UP:

Add a challenge to this move by holding the position for five seconds after raising up on the balls of your feet, then slowly lower back down.

Take Care
Don't lean forward as you raise up but keep your back straight.

SEE IT: bodylastics.com/exercise/standing-calf-raises-with-flat-bands

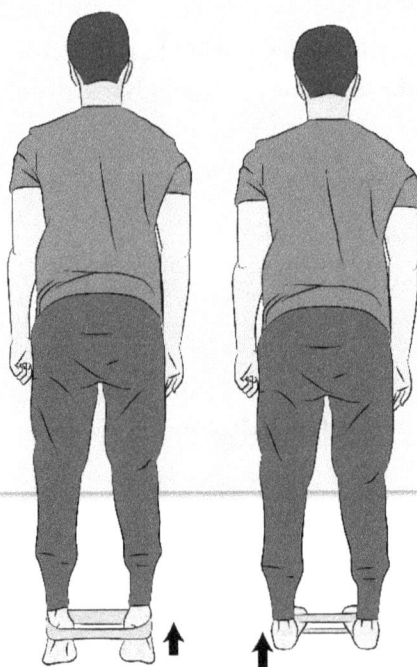

STANDING CALF RAISE WITH MINI BAND

BAND USED: MINI BAND | **TIME NEEDED:** 3 MINUTES

DIRECTIONS:

1. Loop the mini band around both feet with the band touching the front of your ankles and under the back of your heels. Stand with your feet hip-width distance apart or until the band is taut.
2. Inhale as you raise up onto the balls of your feet while keeping your core tight to maintain balance. Exhale as you reach the top of the move, then inhale as you lower your heels back down to the starting position. This is one rep.

3. Do 15 reps for 3 sets.

LEVEL UP:

To strengthen calves even more, hold the position at the top of the move for five seconds, then slowly lower your heels back down to the floor.

Take Care
If this challenges your balance, hold on to a countertop or a sturdy chair to steady yourself. This move can also be done seated. You can add weight to the tops of your thighs while seated if needed.

SEE IT: livestrong.com/article/103743-resistance-band-calf-exercises

Part 3
The Action
Plan

Chapter 8:
Three-Week Program
for Beginners

W e have come to the exciting part of putting these exercises into action! In this chapter, there is a program for three weeks for beginners or those just getting into strength training for the first time or after having been away from it for a while. Strength training should not be done every day. Remember, rest and recovery are just as important for muscles as strength training. During training, muscles experience fatigue and micro-tears that are necessary for them to repair, build, and grow. On your rest days or days where you work different muscles, the fatigued muscles get a chance to recover.

Highlights of this three-week program include

- strength training two days a week. Leave two or three days in between strength training days where you do other exercises such as walking, bike riding, swimming, or playing a sport.
- planning on about 30 minutes of strength training on each scheduled day.
- as a beginner or someone getting back into exercising, paying attention to your body and any muscle soreness. There will be some soreness, but you should not feel pain.
- continuing on this beginner program for as long as you need to until you are comfortable advancing to the intermediate program.

Week One

It's your first week, so take it slow and easy. Learn to do the move correctly and don't worry about how quickly you are working.

Day 1

- **Biceps and triceps:** bicep curl, crossbow triceps extension
- **Chest and back:** chest punch, pull apart
- **Core and glutes:** bridge, clamshell
- **Quads and hamstrings:** banded leg extension, band pull through
- **Forearms and calves:** behind the back wrist curl, ankle pumps
-

Day 2

- **Biceps and triceps:** lying hammer curl, overhead triceps extension
- **Chest and back:** crossover fly, reverse fly
- **Core and glutes:** double leg stretch, scissor toe tap
- **Quads and hamstrings:** curtsy squat, bird dog

- **Forearms and calves:** forearm curl, marches with calf raise

Week Two

This week there are no new exercises as you will be doing what you did last week. However, you will now concentrate on flexing and squeezing your muscles as you work them to get the most out of these moves. Master them because next week we will introduce some new moves!

Day 1

- **Biceps and triceps:** bicep curl, crossbow triceps extension
- **Chest and back:** chest punch, pull apart
- **Core and glutes:** bridge, clamshell
- **Quads and hamstrings:** banded leg extension, band pull through
- **Forearms and calves:** behind the back wrist curl, ankle pumps

Day 2

- **Biceps and triceps:** lying hammer curl, overhead triceps extension
- **Chest and back:** crossover fly, reverse fly
- **Core and glutes:** double leg stretch, scissor toe tap
- **Quads and hamstrings:** curtsy squat, bird dog
- **Forearms and calves:** forearm curl, marches with calf raise

Week Three

New exercises are introduced this week! Notice how folding in these new exercises challenges your muscles in a different way.

Day 1

- **Biceps and triceps:** reverse bicep curl, triceps kickback
- **Chest and back:** lying chest press, seated row
- **Core and glutes:** mountain climber, side steps
- **Quads and hamstrings:** deadlift, good mornings
- **Forearms and calves:** rear rotation, standing calf raise with flat band

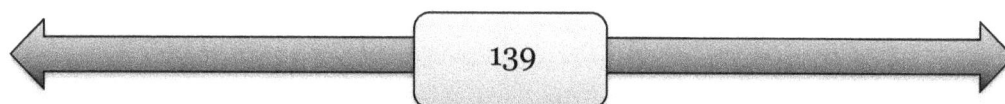

Day 2

- **Biceps and triceps:** single arm hammer curl, triceps shoulder press
- **Chest and back:** pullover, standing Y
- **Core and glutes:** pall of press, squats
- **Quads and hamstrings:** lying leg press, lying leg curl
- **Forearms and calves:** reverse forearm curl, standing calf raise with mini band

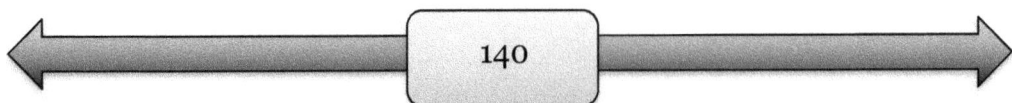

Chapter 9
Three-Week Program
For Intermediate

Now that you are back into exercising regularly and are slowly building strength, you are ready to move on to a more challenging program for intermediate exercisers! Remember that no matter what level you are currently at, strength training should not be done on the same muscles every day. Muscles need time to rest and recover in order for them to grow and strengthen.

Highlights of this intermediate three-week program include

- strength training remains at two days a week. Incorporate some cardio in between your strength training days. It doesn't have to be just walking on a treadmill. Include some fun cardio like dancing, cross-country skiing, or hiking.
- planning on about 40 minutes of strength training on your scheduled days.
- not being afraid of dropping back into the beginner routine every other week if you find yourself getting overwhelmed at the intermediate level. Pay attention to your body and how it feels after you exercise.

Week One

This week, we will slowly add an extra exercise to a few of the muscle groups. On Day 1, there is one extra exercise for the biceps/triceps, core/glutes, and forearms/calves. Then on Day 2, there is one extra exercise in the chest/back and quads/hamstrings categories. This should only add 10 minutes of time to your workout.

Day 1

- **Biceps and triceps:** reverse bicep curl, bicep curl, triceps kickback
- **Chest and back:** lying chest press, seated row
- **Core and glutes:** mountain climber, bridge, side steps
- **Quads and hamstrings:** deadlift, good mornings
- **Forearms and calves:** rear rotation, behind the back wrist curl, standing calf raise with flat band

Day 2

- **Biceps and triceps:** single arm hammer curl, triceps shoulder press
- **Chest and back:** pullover, chest punch, standing Y
- **Core and glutes:** pall of press, squats
- **Quads and hamstrings:** lying leg press, banded leg extension, lying leg curl

- **Forearms and calves:** reverse forearm curl, standing calf raise with mini band

Week Two

Are you feeling it? The added exercises are meant to be a little more challenging now that you are getting stronger and more accustomed to resistance training.

Day 1

- **Biceps and triceps:** bicep curl, crossbow triceps extension, triceps kickback
- **Chest and back:** chest punch, pull apart
- **Core and glutes:** bridge, clamshell, side steps
- **Quads and hamstrings:** banded leg extension, band pull through
- **Forearms and calves:** behind the back wrist curl, ankle pumps, standing calf raise with flat band

Day 2

- **Biceps and triceps:** lying hammer curl, overhead triceps extension
- **Chest and back:** crossover fly, reverse fly, seated row
- **Core and glutes:** double leg stretch, scissor toe tap
- **Quads and hamstrings:** curtsy squat, bird dog, good mornings
- **Forearms and calves:** forearm curl, marches with calf raise

Week Three

Now that you are used to these added exercises, really concentrate on your form and you're breathing this week. Be sure to squeeze and flex the muscle you are working for the mind-body exercise connection.

Day 1

- **Biceps and triceps:** reverse bicep curl, lying hammer curl, overhead triceps extension
- **Chest and back:** lying chest press, reverse fly
- **Core and glutes:** mountain climber, double leg stretch, clamshell
- **Quads and hamstrings:** deadlift, band pull through
- **Forearms and calves:** rear rotation, forearm curl, ankle pumps

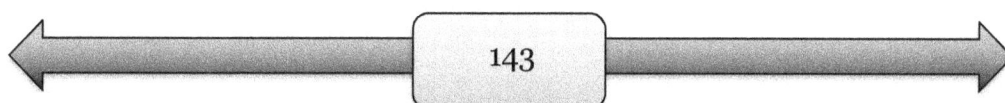

Day 2

- **Biceps and triceps:** single arm hammer curl, crossbow triceps extension
- **Chest and back:** pullover, crossover fly, standing Y
- **Core and glutes:** pall of press, squats
- **Quads and hamstrings:** lying leg press, curtsy squat, lying leg curl
- **Forearms and calves:** reverse forearm curl, standing calf raise with mini band

Chapter 10
Three-Week Program
for Advanced

You are doing great, and you've made it to this advanced level of resistance training! It doesn't matter how many months it has taken you to get here; the fact is you have been consistent in your resistance band workouts and are ready for something more challenging. Just because you are now accustomed to working out doesn't mean you throw away beginner and intermediate workout programs. You can still use those! Fold them into your weeks whenever you want to change things up. Remember, your muscles benefit from being surprised.

Highlights of this three-week program for advanced exercisers include

- strength training increases to three days a week. Don't worry if this sounds overwhelming. It's not!
- exercises are split up differently so that you will be working the upper body and lower body on alternate days. One week, you will work the upper body twice that week and the following week you will work the lower body twice.
- workout sessions are between 30 and 40 minutes, depending on the day.

Week One

This week you will be concentrating on the upper body and working it twice this week while working the lower body just once. Remember to include a cardio day or rest day between these strength training days.

Day 1 Upper Body

- **Biceps and triceps:** bicep curl, lying hammer curl, crossbow triceps extension, overhead triceps extension
- **Chest and back:** chest punch, crossover fly, pull apart, reverse fly
- **Forearms:** behind the back wrist curl, forearm curl

Day 2 Lower Body

- **Core and glutes:** bridge, double leg stretch, clamshell, scissor toe tap
- **Quads and hamstrings:** banded leg extension, curtsy squat, band pull through, bird dog
- **Calves:** ankle pumps, standing calf raise with flat band

Day 3 Upper Body

- Biceps and triceps: reverse bicep curl, single arm hammer curl, triceps kickback, triceps shoulder press
- Chest and back: lying chest press, pullover, seated row, standing Y
- Forearms: rear rotation, reverse forearm curls

Week Two

It is your lower body's turn this week to be worked out twice. Your upper body is only being worked out once, so it's a good week to play tennis or ping-pong. And it's always a good week to include dance as your cardio!

Day 1 Lower Body

- **Core and glutes:** mountain climber, pall of press, side step, squats
- **Quads and hamstrings:** deadlift, lying leg press, good mornings, lying leg curl
- **Calves:** marches with calf raise, standing calf raise with mini band

Day 2 Upper Body

- **Biceps and triceps:** bicep curl, lying hammer curl, crossbow triceps extension, overhead triceps extension
- **Chest and back:** chest punch, crossover fly, pull apart, reverse fly
- **Forearms:** behind the back wrist curl, forearm curl

Day 3 Lower Body

- **Core and glutes:** bridge, double leg stretch, clamshell, scissor toe tap
- **Quads and hamstrings:** banded leg extension, curtsy squat, band pull through, bird dog
- **Calves:** ankle pumps, standing calf raise with flat band

Week Three

Are you seeing a pattern here? The upper body is being worked on twice this week and the lower body just once.

Day 1 Upper Body

- **Biceps and triceps:** bicep curl, reverse bicep curl, crossbow triceps extension, triceps kickback
- **Chest and back:** chest punch, lying chest press, pull apart, reverse fly
- **Forearms:** forearm curl, reverse forearm curl

Day 2 Lower Body

- **Core and glutes:** mountain climber, pall of press, side step, squats
- **Quads and hamstrings:** deadlift, lying leg press, good mornings, lying leg curl
- **Calves:** marches with calf raise, standing calf raise with mini band

Day 3 Upper Body

- **Biceps and triceps:** lying hammer curl, single arm hammer curl, overhead triceps extension, triceps shoulder press
- **Chest and back:** crossover fly, pullover, seated row, standing Y
- **Forearms:** behind the back wrist curl, rear rotation

Conclusion

Congratulations!

You have completed reading through this book and we hope you have learned how to get on the road to better health after 60. It can be done! One of the goals in putting this guide together was to give people a road map and the tools needed to start or restart their strength training workouts.

We've covered a lot of information in this book. The main sections were broken down into three parts: the foundation, the exercises, and the action plan. The foundation chapters provided information, tips, and a few things to think over such as goals and motivation. The exercise chapters outlined exercises for different areas of the body and included the how-tos, the precautions, and an online video link to view how the exercise is performed correctly. Finally, in the action plan, we put it all together in three different workout programs specifically for beginners, intermediate, and advanced exercisers.

Some takeaways from Chapters 1 and 2 included the following:

- You can maintain and build bone density as well as gain muscle strength with resistance band exercises.
- Resistance bands are an ideal piece of workout equipment because they are inexpensive, lightweight, easy to store, and adaptable to all levels of fitness.
- There are many types of resistance bands. Flat bands can be loop bands, mini bands, or therapy bands. Tubular bands include figure 8 bands or tube bands with handles.
- Good form and proper breathing are important for getting the most out of the exercises. Common mistakes are easily avoided.
- Putting together a workout program is easy once you've defined your goal and identified the exercises needed to help you achieve that goal.

In Chapter 3, we explored exercises for the main muscles in your upper arm, the biceps and triceps. The bones and muscles here are important for helping you to perform daily tasks such as opening doors, pushing drawers closed, and hugging grandkids.
The chest and back muscles were emphasized in Chapter 4. These muscles assist your lungs to expand and your spine to stay erect. Having a strong chest and back also keeps your upper body stable as you carry grocery bags, lift items, and open jars or bottles.

We learned about the necessity of strong core and glute muscles in Chapter 5. This is a chapter that is a must for older adults because of the role that the core and glute muscles play in the balance, flexibility, and stability of the whole body.

In Chapter 6, we looked at the quads and hamstrings. These large muscles in your thighs are all-important in their function to help us sit, stand, jump, and walk. To remain independent and able to do basic tasks, we need to train these muscles.

The forearms and calves don't get a lot of attention, but we devoted Chapter 7 to these smaller muscles of our extremities. These muscles are gateways to the strength of the whole limbs. We need strong forearms to support the rest of our arms as well as solid calves to reinforce our entire legs.

Once we learned about the variety of exercises that can be done with resistance bands, it was time to put them into action! Chapter 8 included a three-week exercise program tailored for beginners. For those who are just starting on their exercise journey, or for those who are recovering from illness or injury and getting back into working out, this chapter took things slow and easy with two workouts a week. Each day included a full-body workout that hit all areas from head to toe.

In Chapter 9, there was a three-week program for those ready to move on to the intermediate level. Workouts were kept at two days a week, but additional exercises were added to slightly increase the time spent on strength training. It is also recommended to add cardio on the days that strength training is not performed. Cardio can be anything from biking to walking, cross-country skiing to hiking, or dancing to walking upstairs.

Finally, in Chapter 10 we arrived at the advanced level of the program! This chapter is for those who are ready for a challenge. In the advanced workouts, the number of days a week increased to three times. Exercises were divided up into upper body focused or lower body focused and done on alternating scheduled days. As mentioned, the beginner and intermediate programs aren't discarded but can still be incorporated into weeks where the reader may have less time or energy.

Here we are at the end. It has been a wonderful journey teaching you about the effectiveness and ease of resistance band training. My hope and prayer is that you will not only have gained knowledge in this area, but will put into practice what you have learned. You have the tools and the know-how, now it is decision time to actually do it. If this book has helped you, we'd love to hear about it! Please consider leaving a comment or review online. Your words have the potential to make a real difference, not just to me, but also to those who may discover my work in the future. I'm proud of you and wish you the best as you grow in age and in health.

Scan the QR code:

I hope you enjoy good health and happiness on the long road ahead of you, and I wish you all the best. Thank you for allowing me to share my knowledge with you.

Baz Thompson

References

1. Akram, M. (2022, March 5). *7 best resistance band quad exercises for sturdy legs.* Fitness Phantom. https://thefitnessphantom.com/resistance-band-quad-exercises

2. Capritto, A., & Galic, B. (2023, March 7). The only 5 resistance band exercises older adults need for healthy aging. Livestrong. https://www.livestrong.com/article/108869-resistance-band-exercises-seniors/

3. Bodylastics. (2023a, March 20). *One arm overhead triceps extension with bands.* Bodylastics. https://bodylastics.com/exercise/one-arm-overhead-triceps-extension-with-bands/

4. Bodylastics. (2023b, March 21). *Lying hammer curl (arms down) with bands.* Bodylastics. https://bodylastics.com/exercise/lying-hammer-curl-with-bands-arms-down/

5. Bodylastics. (2023c, March 29). *Standing calf raises with flat resistance bands.* Bodylastics. https://bodylastics.com/exercise/standing-calf-raises-with-flat-bands/

6. Centers for Disease Control and Prevention. (2020). *Disability impacts all of us infographic.* Centers for Disease Control and Prevention. https://www.cdc.gov/ncbddd/disabilityandhealth/infographic-disability-impacts-all.html

7. Cleveland Clinic. (2022, May 4). How effective are resistance bands for strength training? Cleveland Clinic. https://health.clevelandclinic.org/should-you-try-resistance-bands-for-strength-training/

8. Clifton, T. (2021, June 25). *Resistance band workouts for abs: 11 exercises to trys.* Healthline. https://www.healthline.com/health/fitness/resistance-band-workouts-abs

9. Coach Sofia. (2020, May 9). *5 resistance band hamstrings exercises (do these at home!).* Coach Sofia Fitness. https://www.coachsofiafitness.com/5-resistance-band-hamstrings-exercises-do-these-at-home/

10. Coleman, S. (2021a, April 15). *6 resistance band bicep exercises & workouts for bigger arms.* Set for Set. https://www.setforset.com/blogs/news/bicep-exercises-and-workouts-with-resistance-bands

11. Coleman, S. (2021b, April 18). *6 best resistance band tricep exercises for all three heads.* Set for Set. https://www.setforset.com/blogs/news/resistance-band-tricep-exercises

12. Davis, N. (2021, June 9). *10 back exercises with bands to counteract work-from-home posture.* Healthline. https://www.healthline.com/health/fitness/back-exercises-with-bands#Exercises-to-combat-work-from-home-posture

13. Edwards, T. (2021, May 6). *Resistance band chest workout: 7 exercises you can do anywhere.* Healthline. https://www.healthline.com/health/fitness/resistance-band-chest-workout#exercises

14. Eisinger, A. (2019, November 19). *6 effective exercises that really work your butt.* Self. https://www.self.com/gallery/5-effective-resistance-band-exercises-for-a-strong-firm-butt

15. Fetters, K. A. (2022, March 29). *The total-body resistance band workout.* SilverSneakers. https://www.silversneakers.com/blog/total-body-resistance-band-workout-older-adults/

16. Free Trainers. (2023, March 26). *Bands lying chest press.* Free Trainers. https://www.freetrainers.com/exercise/exercise/bands_lying_chest_press/

17. Freytag, C. (2021, October 7). How learning good form can help your strength training. Verywell Fit. https://www.verywellfit.com/basic-strength-training-tips-for-good-form-3498161

18. Freytag, C. (2023a, March 21). *How to do resistance band push-ups.* Get Healthy U. https://gethealthyu.com/exercise/resistance-band-push/

19. Freytag, C. (2023b, March 21). *How to do resistance band tricep shoulder press.* Get Healthy U. https://gethealthyu.com/exercise/resistance-band-tricep-shoulder-press/

20. Galic, B. (2020, June 25). *The only 5 resistance band exercises you need for toned calves.* Livestrong. https://www.livestrong.com/article/103743-resistance-band-calf-exercises/

21. Holzbaur, K. R. S., Murray, W. M., Gold, G. E., & Delp, S. L. (2007). Upper limb muscle volumes in adult subjects. *Journal of Biomechanics, 40*(4), 742–749. https://doi.org/10.1016/j.jbiomech.2006.11.011

22. Hong, A. R., & Kim, S. W. (2018). Effects of resistance exercise on bone health. *Endocrinology and Metabolism, 33*(4), 435–444. https://doi.org/10.3803/enm.2018.33.4.435

23. Jackson, J. (2022, May 2). *Resistance band forearm exercises and workouts for muscle growth.* Critical Body. https://criticalbody.com/resistance-band-forearm-exercises/

24. Liu, X., Gao, Y., Lu, J., Ma, Q., Shi, Y., Liu, J., Xin, S., & Su, H. (2022). Effects of different resistance exercise forms on body composition and muscle strength in overweight and/or obese individuals: A systematic review and meta-analysis. *Frontiers in Physiology, 12.* https://doi.org/10.3389/fphys.2021.791999

25. Lopes, J. S. S., Machado, A. F., Micheletti, J. K., de Almeida, A. C., Cavina, A. P., & Pastre, C. M. (2019). Effects of training with elastic resistance versus conventional resistance on muscular strength: A systematic review and meta-analysis. *SAGE Open Medicine, 7*, 205031211983111. https://doi.org/10.1177/2050312119831116

26. Migala, J. (2022, April 13). *How to use resistance bands: For absolute beginners.* Everyday Health. https://www.everydayhealth.com/fitness/how-to-get-started-with-resistance-band-workouts-an-absolute-beginners-guide/

27. Silver Sneakers [@silversneakerseditors7401]. (2023a, March 25). *Resistance band biceps curl* [Video]. YouTube. https://youtu.be/LI1p31gp_fU

28. Silver Sneakers [@silversneakerseditors7401]. (2023b, March 25). *Resistance band chest punch* [Video]. YouTube. https://youtu.be/SYVotAbHHpE

29. Silver Sneakers [@silversneakerseditors7401]. (2023c, March 25). *Seated row with resistance band* [Video]. YouTube. https://youtu.be/6bvCuSeXLwc

30. Morrisey, P. (2023, March 26). *How to do: Band tricep kickback.* Skimble. https://www.skimble.com/exercises/57597-band-tricep-kickback-how-to-do-exercise

31. Stepanov, P. (2023, March 26). *Hammer curl with a resistance band - expert tips, and mistakes to avoid.* Hevy. https://www.hevyapp.com/exercises/hammer-curl-resistance-band/

32. U.S. Department of Health and Human Services. (2018). *Physical activity guidelines for Americans 2nd edition.* Health.gov https://health.gov/sites/default/files/201909/Physical_Activity_Guidelines_2nd_edition.pdf

33. West Bend Staff. (2023, March 20). *Resistance band safety.* The Silver Lining. https://www.thesilverlining.com/safety-tips/resistance-band-safety

Image References

1. Alenius, G. (2019, March 10). *Fitness girl working out outdoors with loop band* [Photo]. Unsplash. https://unsplash.com/photos/rG3N_CXMeio?utm_source=unsplash&utm_medium=referral&utm_content=creditShareLink

2. Sikkema, K. (2018, January 12). *It's more fun to take pictures of fitness equipment than to use it* [Photo]. Unsplash. https://unsplash.com/photos/rWBBDErPXcY?utm_source=unsplash&utm_medium=referral&utm_content=creditShareLink